LATENCY
The Golden Age of Childhood

Psychoanalytical Developmental Theory
According to Freud, Klein and Bion

Gertraud Diem-Wille

Translated by Benjamin McQuade

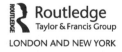

Routledge
Taylor & Francis Group

LONDON AND NEW YORK

First published in German in 2015 as
*Latenz—Das "goldene Zeitalter" der Kindheit Psychoanalytische
Entwicklungstheorie nach Freud, Klein und Bion*
by W. Kohlhammer GmbH

First published in English in 2018
by Routledge
2 Park Square, Milton Park, Abingdon, Oxon OX14 4RN

and by Routledge
711 Third Avenue, New York, NY 10017

Routledge is an imprint of the Taylor & Francis Group, an informa business

British Library Cataloguing-in-Publication Data
A catalogue record for this book is available from the British Library

Library of Congress Cataloging-in-Publication Data
A catalog record has been requested for this book

ISBN-13: 978-1-78220-543-2 (pbk)

Typeset in Palatino
by V Publishing Solutions Pvt Ltd., Chennai, India

LATENCY

CONTENTS

ABOUT THE AUTHOR

Gertraud Diem-Wille is professor of psychoanalysis in education at the University of Klagenfurt, in southern Austria. She is a training analyst for children, adolescents, and adults of the Viennese Psychoanalytic Society and the International Psychoanalytical Association (IPA). She has pioneered and supported the training in psychoanalytic observational approaches to training in psychoanalysis and in educational fields. She is the organising and scientific tutor of the postgraduate master's degree course in psychoanalytic observational studies at the University of Klagenfurt. Her books include *Young Children and their Parents: Perspectives from Psychoanalytic Infant Observation* (Karnac, 2014) and *The Early Years of Life: Psychoanalytical Development Theory According to Freud, Klein, and Bion* (Karnac, 2011).

INTRODUCTION

The period of a child's life between six and eleven years of age brings major changes. The toddler becomes a schoolchild, who must find his place in a new group as part of compulsory participation in school. Children must also learn cultural techniques, alongside their introduction to reading and writing.

It may seem curious that psychoanalysis treats this eventful period in such a neglectful fashion. We can search in vain for relevant psychoanalytic books on this phase of life, which Freud called the latency period. Moreover, the concept itself has hardly entered everyday usage. There are presumably two reasons for this. First, Freud assumed that the foundation for personality development is laid in the first six years of life, where sexual core identity is developed and the basic patterns of the personality are established. Certainly, these basic patterns can be altered, but they remain embedded at the deepest level. The second reason is linked to Freud's concept of libidinal development. After the early intense years of Oedipal wishes and conflicts, libidinous desires now retreat to the background since the Oedipal conflict itself has retreated—these wishes are only *latent*, exhibiting themselves less obviously. Only in puberty does drive development reawaken, erupting with a tempestuous force that propels new forms of psychic development.

The latency phase serves to bind these two volatile periods together, and consequently does not receive central attention.

This relatively tranquil period, where libidinal development is put on the back burner, is the time every society appropriates for children to start school—the time of "scholastic readiness". At this age, children's interest is no longer fixed on their bodies or their parents' bodies, but on the outer world and their school friends or teachers. They wish to acquire knowledge that will allow them a new kind of independence. They begin to go to school alone, read signs and simple texts, and thus take in information in a more independent fashion. This is why Freud writes of the "golden time of childhood": for that matter, this period is relatively pleasant for teachers and parents, and relatively conflict-free (compared to the period preceding it). The ship of child development, after the storms of the early years, now navigates through relatively calm waters. Children enjoy doing things together with their parents. Activities such as hiking, swimming, boating, going to the cinema, or making music together are popular.

What remains from early childhood is the great individual difference between children, who manifest their inborn temperaments and react to situations within a given family and its social context. This latency phase reveals whether parents and children have succeeded in laying the basis for a beneficial, positive emotional development. Inadequately mastered inner conflicts—manifested in fears of monsters, spiders, giants, or dogs—can now retreat to the background.

Children vary in how they choose to take leave of the phase of early childhood. Stefanie wishes a "last doll" for herself, Sebastian wants a "real fishing rod" now, in order to prepare for the challenges of the angler's licence test. Some things children earlier desired eagerly they now see as "babyish" and reject scornfully.

CHAPTER ONE

Body and psyche in latency

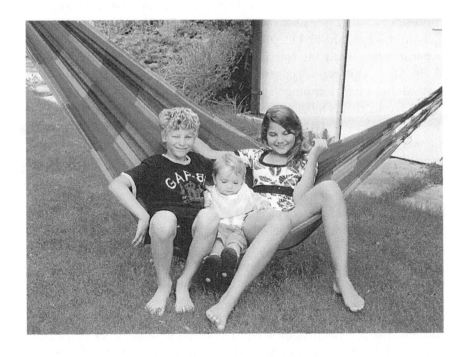

The body ego

After the first years of dramatic physical development in a child's life, the subsequent period of latency (six to twelve years old) represents a time of emotional and physical stabilisation. The newborn infant's body, with its limited means of communication, vision, and smell, had developed rapidly into a baby who could raise his hands over his head, stamp, hold his toes, and turn over. Parents enthuse over their baby's developing skills as he crawls, sits, or stands up, and begins to walk. Anyone following the progress of an invalid who once again must "learn" to walk knows how difficult it is for limbs to again become limber, regain balance, and embark on the task of walking. Yet a small child develops these skills easily through playful experimentation—fuelled simply by his desire for mobility. Each child has his own rhythm and dynamic process culminating in standing up and walking. The child's world is indeed many-faceted, as can be seen in close examination through systematic psychoanalytic observation in play groups or the family; these psychoanalytic observations are subsequently described by the observer, who analyses them for their relevance regarding the child's personality (see Diem-Wille & Turner, 2012).

From his hesitant first steps, the baby becomes a mobile, vital child experimenting with his steadily increasing mobility and movement skills. At six, children are constantly in motion: they in fact rarely walk, instead hopping, jumping, running, and climbing—with, as Anna Freud wrote, their *Funktionslust*, "pleasure in functioning", that is, the desire and pleasure to have their bodies under control. Toilet training already constitutes an important accomplishment, requiring control over the sphincter muscles. At first, releasing bodily products was an act bound up in the baby's relationship with the mother: submitting the stool is symbolically linked to giving the mother a gift, and in a struggle between child and mother, the child's desire to retain the stool can lead to contretemps. Thus, both releasing and submitting are steps towards maturity.

Psyche and soma are intimately linked. In this section, I observe the child's development from the somatic point of view—although the psychic level must always be taken into consideration. The way a child experiences her own body depends upon what has happened to her and how her parents treat their child's body—whether or not they contemplate it lovingly, caress and care for it in joy and gladness over the child's existence. Such a lovingly contemplated child will feel well in his own skin—"cathecting" (occupying) his body positively, in Freud's terminology—and regard his body as do his loving parents, experiencing himself as something vital. When parents are in a difficult situation and cannot devote themselves lovingly to their baby, if they are overwhelmed by their own problems and caring for the baby becomes merely a matter of duty, their child consequently cannot "cathect" his body in a positive fashion: instead, he feels himself a stranger within his own skin, or avoids bodily contact with others.

The subsequent chapters focus on the development of feeling, thinking, and psychosexual development—as closely interlinked as in a symphony, where various instruments determine together the tonal colour. One could also say that the body is a mirror of the soul. Psychic blocks, guilt feelings, and fears are manifested through clumsy movements, frequent bruises, and inhibited forms of expression. An emotionally secure child with a good relationship to her parents moves with security and ease. She shows her lust for life by not just walking but jumping, estimating her own capabilities realistically and only climbing up where she can subsequently climb down. The inherent potential every child has for physical development can be tapped when parents trust their children to follow their inner programme for development. Here, it suffices for parents to be emotionally accessible, showing their joy and involvement with the child's development—for instance, simply paying attention while he learns to crawl or stand up. Emmi Pikler (2001), a Hungarian paediatrician with psychoanalytic experience, strongly advises affording a child time, not overambitiously forcing him to acquire a skill (for instance, sitting or walking) before he has developed the requisite muscles. The psychoanalytic theory of development correlates with this basic attitude, emphasising in turn the underlying emotional quality of the parent–child relationship—particularly the parent's capacity for absorbing and understanding the child's primitive fears as projected into the parent, subsequently explaining those fears to the child in easily comprehensible language. In addition, the parents' positive expectations that their child will indeed develop the necessary capabilities will furnish a positive influence. Overly fearful, unconsciously aggressive parents who constantly expect their child to hurt himself, have an accident, or fail can have an inhibiting influence. Psychoanalysis attempts to detect unconscious, suppressed feelings and motives behind parents' manifest behaviour and feelings. We know that there are always ambivalent feelings within human relationships, that the baby can feel love and hate for the same sheltering person from whom she also desires independence. If parents are able to perceive the dark side of their relationship to their child, this can actually constitute a relief. Mother and father recognise that alongside their love for the child, they in fact desire to again be alone together in peace, at times experiencing the child as an intruder into their private intimacy.

We understand the body ego on the one hand as a medium for communication; movement expresses psychic and emotional moods, activities, and inhibitions. On the other hand, it is also of essential import how a person—whether child or adult—has emotionally cathected his body. The way a person feels his own body is a result of his original, primary relationship to his parents. When a child sees the "shine" in his mother's eyes (as D. W. Winnicott put it), expressing her delight over his existence, he will accordingly build up a positive feeling towards his body and self and feel comfortable in his skin. "The ego is first and foremost a bodily ego; it is not merely a surface entity, but is itself the projection of a surface," as Freud wrote in *The Ego and the Id* (1923b, p. 294). In a footnote to the English translation, Freud adds: "The ego is ultimately derived from bodily sensations, chiefly from those springing from the surface of the body. It may thus be regarded as a mental projection of the surface of the body, besides as we have seen above, representing the superficies of the mental apparatus" (ibid.). The way we psychically cathect our bodies depends upon our self-image: can we perceive our body as belonging to us, or does it remain something foreign like a robot or mechanical machine? In my book *The Early Years of Life* (2013), I described the basic aspects of body cathexis as a reflection of the emotional relationship to the primary caregiver—when the child feels accepted, expected, and loved, or when he interprets his parents' devotion, denial, joy, and irritation within his own fantasy world. We understand the child's bodily self-image—and his acceptance of this self-image—as an internalisation of his experiences when his parents have treated his body either lovingly or dismissively. Although the complex interrelations between self-image, self-consciousness, and acceptance of the body are treated in separate chapters of this book, it must be emphasised that these various perspectives always overlap.

In the latency period between six and twelve years of age (the temporal definition of latency varies, beginning with either five or six and proceeding to eleven or twelve), the child's peer group focuses

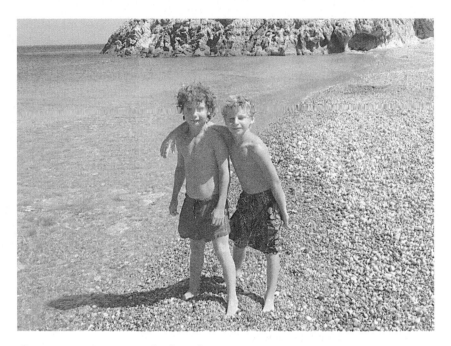

Illustration 1: Boys on the beach.

on the acquirement of physical skills. Freud adopted his concept of "latency" from Wilhelm Fliess, who spoke of the "period of sexual latency". Freud understands latency as a transition between early childhood and adolescence, bridging these two periods. Here, the term "latency" denotes that sexual ambitions are not as obvious as in the Oedipal phase or in adolescence, remaining relatively occluded. In his *Three Essays on the Theory of Sexuality*, Freud posits that the energy from sexual impulses "is diverted, wholly or in great part, from their sexual use and directed to other ends" (1905d, p. 178). All of the child's prior experiences, her inhibitions, fantasies, and desires have already served to form the basic pattern of her personality, remaining immanent throughout her lifetime. Although they will be modified through later experiences, the deep structures remain constant. In latency, however, sexual impulses become subordinated to other goals.

The acquirement of bodily skills moves to the forefront. One biological manifestation of maturity is the loss of baby teeth and the growing in of "adult" teeth—an event children yearn for, impatiently wiggling their teeth at the slightest evidence of looseness. Now, the child shifts from infantile aggressions to more constructive activities.

Freud points out that "children feel a need for a large amount of active muscular exercise and derive extraordinary pleasure from satisfying it" (ibid., p. 202). This is borne out by the following poem by A. A. Milne:

> *Hoppity*
>
> Christopher Robin goes
> Hoppity, hoppity,
>
> Hoppity, hoppity, hop.
> Whenever I tell him
> Politely to stop it, he
> Says he can't possibly stop.
>
> If he stopped hopping,
> He couldn't go anywhere,
> Poor little Christopher
> Couldn't go anywhere …
> That's why he always goes
> Hoppity, hoppity,
> Hoppity,
> Hoppity,
> Hop.
>
> (*When We Were Very Young*, 1924, pp. 60ff.)

Hopping and running are expressions of the child's overflowing joy in life. He cannot help moving in this mode, taking pleasure in a new-found control over his own body, exercising his new skills.

With tremendous perseverance and stamina, the child proceeds through all manner of skilled games and sports: cycling, skateboarding, climbing, and gymnastics such as cartwheels and handstands, which are sometimes practised for hours on end. Particularly for boys, the measurement of strength, competition, and winning determine social prestige and hierarchical position. Here, the link to sexual pleasure is demonstrated in wrestling and fighting, which can cause sexual excitement as it affords boys considerable body contact in addition to exercising muscles (Freud, 1905d, p. 202).

Boys compete with each other, play wild games, hunt for objects. Action is important (see Brizendine, 2010, p. 39). They fight with swords, toy pistols, water pistols, shouting loudly and attempting to frighten one another. Group games require the capacity to take action and make group decisions. In one popular book for latency children, *Harry Potter* (1997), one game of skill (invented by author J. K. Rowling) is a form of competition: "Quidditch", played on magic broomsticks, imparts to young readers the fascination and physical excitement of flying, embodying an intensified version of popular forms of transportation such as roller skating, skiing, or flying in an aeroplane, plus a strong hint of virtual computer games. With the term "condensation", psychoanalysis understands an essential mechanism found in dreams, where various elements are represented together in a single image (Freud, 1900a, p. 3). As Laplanche and Pontalis describe this mechanism, "A sole idea represents several associative chains at whose point of intersection it is located" (1973, p. 82); Rustin and Rustin (2001, p. 266) note that the magic broomstick is just as much of a status symbol as any other piece of sports equipment—devices children from poorer families cannot afford.

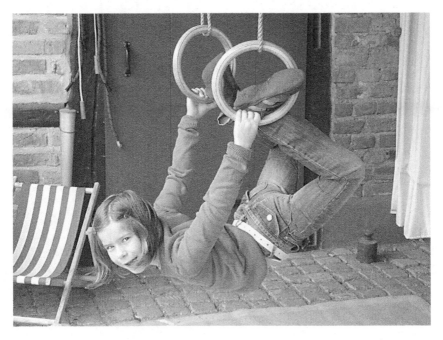

Illustration 2: Girl on the rings.

Brizendine (2006, p. 24) contends that girls dislike rough games: when they are shoved about, they leave the game and seek a quieter corner. Girls also take turns with each other in games of skill "20 times more often than boys" (ibid.); apparently, it is just as important for a girl to watch her friends accomplishing a given feat as accomplishing it herself is. Girls exhibit great persistence in putting together puzzles, drawing, and painting. They also like role-playing—cooking, decorating houses, and caring for dolls. Children's games in latency are more adapted to reality and less rich in fantasy than in early childhood. Melanie Klein (1952c) writes of a "compulsive overemphasis on reality", with attendant repression of fantasy. Whereas small children playing with water express their desire for oral contact and oral dirtying, a child in latency will deal with water in a rationalised form—cooking, cleaning—as expressions of reaction formation, that is, Klein's "compulsive overemphasis on reality".

Clemens, eight, and Katharina, six and a half, are playing "restaurant". Two years before, they played "cooking", making soup out of grass, water, pine needles, and flowers, and serving it to the

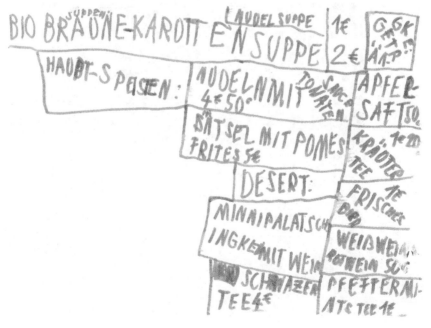

Illustration 3: Menu.

grown-ups out of play bowls. But for latency children, games are much closer to reality: this time, Clemens and Katharina carefully plan a menu, discussing in detail which dishes should be included and how much each will cost. The restaurant's name—"Gasthof zum Attersee"—is written in colourful letters on the menu, and on the other side they draw an Attersee boat. This preparation lasts a full hour, with both children steadily devoting their full concentration to it. They construct a restaurant out of wooden benches where they can cook, then arranging cooking utensils, cutlery, and plates. Now, they approach their parents and other guests, asking what they wish to eat and taking their orders, then returning to the "kitchen" and preparing the dishes ordered. Finally, they serve the dishes, neatly arranged on child plates. When it comes time to pay, they cite a fantasy sum and are somewhat discomfited when the adults pay using leaves, asserting that they would prefer "real money"!

Discussion

This game is strongly characterised by imitation of the adult world. The children slip into the roles of restaurant owners, cook, and waiter. They have already processed their own observations and can represent the

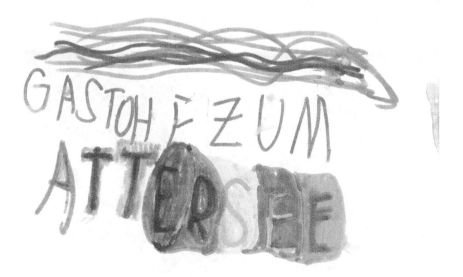

Illustration 4: Restaurant Attersee.

events in a restaurant. There is relatively little room for fantasy, but the game is still fun for both children. Their great energy, and the fact that they repeat the same game the following day, point to a libidinal connection.

That same afternoon, they also invent another game. After swimming and diving for a long time as well as going in an inflatable boat with their mother, they are allowed to play in the boat alone, since it is moored to the wooden pier.

This game, which last for over an hour and is continued the following day, consists of one fixed sequence: both children (who are both good swimmers) are in the boat; Clemens leans far out over the edge, puts his legs in the water, and calls out excitedly: "Man overboard!"; Katharina looks at him in surprise; he (intentionally) slips further and further into the water, as if he were truly falling overboard. Immediately, the girl helps him to get back into the boat—sometimes he manages this alone, sometimes she has to pull him with all her might. She takes up the game, calls out "Man overboard!", and lets herself fall—not as far as Clemens did—into the water. Then she pulls herself out, rolling

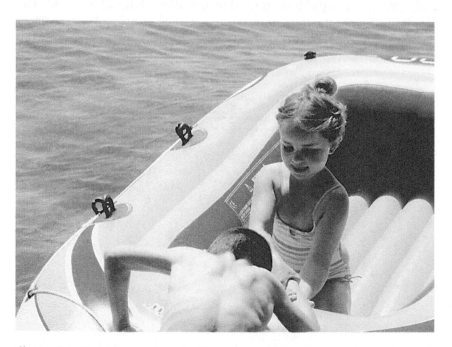

Illustration 5: Man overboard—Woman overboard.

backwards and landing in the bottom of the boat. Each time one of them makes it back into the boat, both children laugh. Katharina then asks why people say "Man overboard" and changes the cry to "Woman overboard". Clemens lands in the boat and plays dead until Katharina brings him back to life.

Then, when both of them wish to go overboard at the same time, the boat capsizes. Clemens is able to swim quickly to the side, but Katharina has her head under the boat, whereupon she swims under it and comes up on the other side. Their mother and grandmother, quickly coming to their aid, help right the boat, and the game continues after a thorough discussion of how to save passengers and a boat when it capsizes.

Discussion

The fun of this game is comprised of various elements. First, it is fascinating for the children to use the boat—a veritable status symbol—without adults. Here, "thrill" (as Michael Balint has put it) is at work—experiencing a limit whose transgression causes both fear and titillation. The children test their powers through a challenging situation, they come into increasing danger, and each saves herself orhimself either alone or with the other's help. Each time, they manage this without any adult help, although security is implicit through the adults' constantly observing them nearby, coming to their aid as soon as serious danger occurs. These children can almost view themselves as adults. Ostensibly by chance, body contact occurs—but this comes under the category of "life-saving", constituting a kind of screen for the pleasant sensations involved.

Some parents become concerned when their child, who previously exhibited a variety of interests, now begins to reiterate the same tasks or games in a seemingly monotonous fashion—as in the case of Monika, who is here described preparing an endless array of little paper rolls:

> Monika comes back from a walk with her grandmother. With a strong sense of purpose, she goes to the cassette recorder and inserts her new Winnie-the-Pooh tape, read by Harry Rowohlt. Listening contentedly, she sits down at her small desk. She takes a ruler, using it to draw lines on a piece of paper until it is filled with lines as broad as the ruler. Then she takes her scissors and slowly

cuts along these lines with an air of great concentration, until she has a series of narrow white strips. Next, she cuts out little pieces of paper on which she writes her name with variously coloured pens. Since she does not yet attend school, she is very proud that she can already write her name correctly. She glues these little nametags onto one strip of paper, in turn gluing the strips of paper together and putting her finished product—which now resembles a napkin ring—onto the dining table. During this, she sings fantasy songs to herself. When her grandmother views and admires her productions, Monika says: "I can't do anything at all, I'm always thinking of new songs I want to sing." When the grandmother tells her to come to eat a snack, she obeys, pushing the pause button and writing the number of the cassette in order to continue with it later. During the snack, Monika's grandmother questions her regarding various sequences from the story—for instance, what each animal gave the donkey Eeyore as a present. Monika answers with great enthusiasm.

Conspicuously and significantly, Monika accomplishes all her activities by herself and without prompting from anyone else. This affords her pleasure, almost as much as if she were an adult fulfilling adult tasks— like her parents sitting at their desk. Drawing with the ruler, cutting the paper with the scissors, pasting on her little nametags all constitute new and rather demanding mechanical skills. Monika produces her handiwork alone, without any help from adults. Yet during this, she is able to take in the contents of the story from the cassette, later describing it when asked to, thus demonstrating she can concentrate on two activities simultaneously. Her perseverance and great enthusiasm are indeed startling, as if she is using absolutely every chance she has to show her grandmother (and herself!) how many things she can do. Monika seems to derive sufficient satisfaction from her grandmother's observing her and occasionally expressing appreciation.

This ritual of repeating the same actions over a greater period of time caused Melanie Klein (1929) to speak of compulsive mechanisms and repression of drive impulses. This terminology is borrowed from pathology, but here signifies an eminently constructive dynamic, where an extended time frame highlights the significance of one special activity.

I understand a child's pleasure in movement and great stamina in sports and fighting to be expressions of healthy narcissism. A positive form of infatuation with one's own body, joy in movement, and feeling pleasurably at home in one's body constitutes a form of narcissism that should not be considered pathological. In his essay "On Narcissism: an Introduction" (1914c), Freud emphasises: "Narcissism in this sense would not be a perversion, but the libidinal complement to the egoism of the instinct of self-preservation, a measure of which may justifiably be attributed to every living creature" (pp. 1–2). Originally, narcissism was understood by P. Näcke—who was quoted by Freud—as a perversion, "the attitude of a person who treats his own body in the same way in which the body of a sexual object is normally treated—who looks at it, that is to say, strokes it and fondles it till he obtains complete satisfaction through these activities" (ibid., p. 1, fn. 1). Freud later discusses the emotional significance of narcissism.

Klein (1948) and Rosenfeld (1987, p. 105) also distinguish between healthy narcissism and the pathological variety. As will be shown in detail in the next chapter, healthy narcissism constitutes the basis of self-worth, not only in the sense of self-idealisation but of self-protection—which is why Rosenfeld employs the term "narcissistic protection".

A short case study will serve to demonstrate the effects of fear and their amelioration through analysis—with light shed particularly on the somatic aspect:

> Fritz, a ten-year-old boy who was sent to therapy due to his social isolation and shyness, entered the therapy room stiffly for his first session. Possessed by fear, he remained in the middle of the room, not daring to even look around it. Only when his fear was described to him as the fear of being with a complete stranger (the therapist) in an unfamiliar room could he sit down on the very edge of a chair, albeit tensely. At first he did not dare to touch anything—not the toys, not the writing and drawing utensils on the table. His serious, prolonged gaze at the pieces of white paper made me interpret that he was perhaps wondering whether he should draw something, and if so, what. Fritz reacted with a surprised look at me. When I added that he might be surprised that I would attempt to understand his thoughts and feelings, he nodded almost imperceptibly and sat in a somewhat more relaxed fashion. At first he seemed completely withdrawn, with his arms folded in front of his body. Towards the end of the hour, he showed me a roll of cough drops and recited an advertising slogan connected to death. When I understood that he was showing me how great his fear of

death was, he relaxed and agreed to come to the second hour. His mother expected him to be able to return home alone after this first session, which I understood as a sign that she in no way understood how frightening it was for him to be together with a new therapist, talking about his inner problems. His mother's behaviour indicates Fritz's emotionally over-challenged state—apparently, she did not understand how important it would be for him to be picked up after the first therapy session: when I questioned her on this, she said she was sure it would be no problem for him, showing how little consideration she had for his emotional rituals.

When, much later—after six months of weekly four-hour analysis—Fritz's intolerable jealousy of his four sisters (born in quick succession after him) became manifest and discussable, his way of using his body began to change. In transference, he demonstrated he wanted to be the only child coming to me for analysis, setting up dangerous traps for the next child (puddles on the floor, turning the water tap so it would spray water on an unsuspecting user). These traps were an alternative to his unconscious guilt feelings over his jealousy and murderous fantasies towards his siblings; he set them traps with pleasure, happy at the thought of how he could trick other children in therapy. He agreed with my interpretations, and became able to show his aggressive desires openly. Fritz attempted—ostensibly by chance—to open the other children's drawers, an unsuccessful attempt since they were locked. He wished to receive more than all the others—wished to take me, my body, and my apartment into his possession. When I made him aware of his hitherto unconscious and forbidden desires, his fear receded and his vitality increased. He saw I understood his desires and aggressive impulses and could, indeed, survive them. His integration of contradictory impulses became manifested in better body skills. He no longer needed to employ his entire energy towards submerging his homicidal unconscious fantasies, but was permitted to feel them; then he became able to show his loving feelings towards his siblings. His surprised parents now reported that Fritz was playing board games with his sisters. He had made friends with the worst-behaved students in his class and they were playing harmless tricks, such as rolling a large snowball down the hill just as girls were approaching. It was impressive to see how sorting out and integrating his contradictory feelings had reduced his inhibitions, thus improving his physical skills. Instead of entering the room with stiff steps, he could now climb from one windowsill to the next; he constructed towering fortresses out of chairs and tables, where he presided as king. He could climb up doorways barefoot and surprised me continually with his physical capabilities. With his parents' approval, he arranged to take part in a course in mountain climbing, in which he participated with great pleasure. Fritz, considered by his mother an "intellectual", only interested in books and never willing to leave his room, had become a boy eager for contact and adventure. Now he could loan the other students his homework and was increasingly respected by them.

Particularly in child analysis, it is continually surprising how strongly the amelioration of fear is manifested somatically. Often, the diminishing of fear and unconscious guilt feelings effects a removal of a somatic blockade, and the child begins to grow, feeling better within his body, developing more self-confidence and cathecting his body positively.

One especially significant rite of passage is the growing of new teeth— an unequivocal sign of the child's graduation into the period of latency and readiness for school. The child greets the first signs of a tooth's loosening with enthusiasm, reporting this phenomenon to everyone at hand. Typically the child starts playfully wiggling her tooth back and forth until it eventually comes out, an event which is duly celebrated.

Sophie, a girl of six and three quarters, called up her grandmother from Sicily, where she was on holiday with her parents. First she told her about the sea, and about the swimming pool with its chemically treated water making it necessary to wear goggles. Then she said dramatically: "Grandma, guess what happened yesterday!" The grandmother was concerned, expecting Sophie to tell of some close call or dangerous situation. But Sophie went on: "Yesterday my second baby tooth fell out!" She then recounted in detail how this had occurred.

This story demonstrates what great emotional significance the transition to permanent, "grown-up" teeth has for the child—a major piece of news to be reported promptly.

Emotional and psychosexual development

Emotional development

The latency child's distanced approach to questions of sex serves to reinforce her personality. As the word "latent" already indicates, Freud assumed that passions here were mainly latent, that is, not in the foreground. The tempestuous phase of Oedipal desires and fears is now succeeded by a calmer phase. The child must collect his strength for a

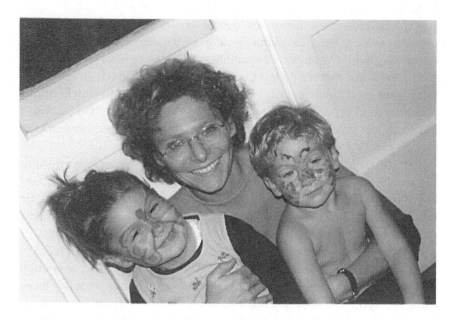

second tempestuous phase—puberty, with its erupting of sexual desires and rapid changes in the body. In latency, interest is directed towards outer reality: play group, school, new friends. Normally, this phase affords the development of an inner identity, which girds the child for her social tasks such as school and the learning of cultural techniques.

Freud described this psychic development in his *Three Essays on the Theory of Sexuality* as follows:

> It is during this period of total or only partial latency that are built up the mental forces which are later to impede the course of the sexual instinct and, like dreams, restrict its flow—disgust, feelings of shame and the aims of aesthetic and moral ideals. (1905d, p. 177)

According to Freud, this development is not caused by education or the child's upbringing, but is "organically based": upbringing and education merely exploit it as a kind of resource.

However, sexual feelings have not completely vanished; instead, the child counters them with the two central defensive mechanisms of latency—reaction formation and sublimation. In the earliest, archaic developmental stage, called the "paranoid-schizoid position" by

Melanie Klein, the defensive mechanism of splitting dominates: this unconscious splitting transforms objects from whole entities into parts of a whole—"part objects". One and the same object's characteristics are transformed into good, idealised part objects on the one hand, and evil, persecuting part objects on the other. Defence mechanisms always operate unconsciously—In later life as well, the splitting mechanism makes other persons be perceived as exclusively good or bad, with their other characteristics ignored (even when plainly visible): for example, we are "blind" to the dark side of someone we love. This tendency towards splitting often occurs in phases of infatuation or intense conflict; after the first phase of being in love, a loved one's unattractive traits, opposing wishes and concepts of life then emerge and a phase of de-idealisation begins, this time with a stronger link to reality. We tend to ascribe our modified assessment not to a better grasp on reality, but instead hold the idealised person responsible for the modification: they have changed, disappointed us, or were previously misrepresenting themselves. The strength of this unconscious splitting mechanism is demonstrated by how crassly we sometimes switch from positive to negative poles, with the admired person suddenly becoming vilified and rejected. Only when the mature form of observation is attained—called the "depressive position" by Melanie Klein—can the observer assume responsibility for previously idealising the object, and positive and negative aspects of *both* members of the relationship can be seen and integrated into a comprehensive image. At this point, a painful modification of the relationship can occur, where positive and negative components are accepted both in the other and in oneself. This constitutes a mature form of relationship where various wishes and needs can be mediated, compromises made, and a certain autonomy within the relationship is possible—constituting a basis not only for happiness and protection, but also for mastering crises and difficulties.

During early development in the first three months of life—the "paranoid-schizoid position" introduced by Melanie Klein—the baby needs help processing his raw sensory perceptions and affects. Bad, dangerous, and primitive sensations are unconsciously projected, with good ones internalised. In this way, the baby protects the good part objects in his mother from his own persecuting, envious, and greedy impulses. Only the mother's capacity for "reverie" or dreamlike empathy (Bion, 1962), or her "primary motherliness" (Winnicott, 1965), enable her to take in these primitive projected feelings. If she is capable of being emotionally touched by these primitive, archaic feelings from her baby, she can then also reflect on them and return them to the baby in an "emotionally digested" form. For example, she might speak with the baby about his fear of death, whereupon the baby ingests ("introjects") these words emotionally; she could say to him, "You're crying as if you might die!" (which also describes the mother's experience of her baby's urgent howling). "You'll get something to eat now, then everything will be fine." Bion believes that it is important for the mother to be truly touched emotionally—to truly feel the fear that the baby projects into her. Through this transformation, called by Bion "the model of container and containment", the baby manages to take these feelings projected into the mother back into himself in the digested form the mother offers. Bion calls the primitive feelings projected by the baby "beta elements" and the feelings as transformed and described verbally by the mother "alpha elements" (see Bion, 1962). A thorough description of this concept can be found in Chapter Two, section 2.2. (I have described the development of thinking in Chapter Four of my book *The Early Years of Life* (2013).)

How the child's feelings develop during latency depends upon whether she can build on an emotionally stable, loving relationship to her mother. If the child has powerful unconscious conflicts and fears, these break through during the latency phase, manifested in problems at school, sleep disorders, extreme shyness, or aggressive, self-destructive behaviour.

Usually, however, this phase of development constitutes a tranquil period after turbulent Oedipal conflicts have been resolved. Identification with the parent of the same sex leads in girls to the wish to be like their mother, and in boys for the wish to be like their father.

There is general agreement that during this period, defence mechanisms undergo a reorganisation, with latency achieving a stability that caused Etchegoyen (1993) to speak of a "theoretical reappraisal". Sarnoff (1976) speaks of a "structure of latency". I shall attempt to describe the state of mind particular to latency, which in some cases can predominate for a person's entire life when further development is blocked.

Defence mechanisms in latency

The psychic processes controlling emotional and psychic events during latency are two defence mechanisms: sublimation and reaction formation. According to Freud, sublimation is "powerful components (...) acquired for every kind of cultural achievement" (1905d, p. 177).

The construction of the unconscious defence forms of sublimation and reaction formation "… probably emerge at the cost of the infantile sexual impulses themselves. Thus the activity of those impulses does not cease even during this period of latency, though their energy is diverted, wholly or in great part, from their sexual use and directed to other ends" (ibid., p. 177). It is important to understand that infantile sexuality always hovers in the background, emerging from time to time and occasionally being expressed in an unexpectedly vehement fashion.

Sublimation

The unconscious defence mechanism "sublimation" is (in Freud) understood to mean a mature form of transferring sexual impulses

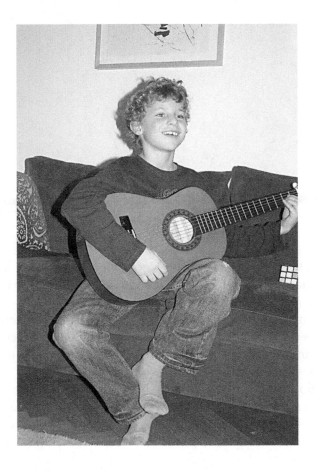

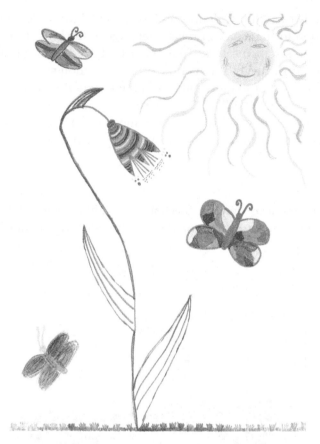

Illustration 6: Drawing by a nine-year-old girl, Katharina: Flower with Sun.

to some other area, consequently achieving satisfaction from this activity. Such activities have no apparent connection to sexuality, but are nevertheless fed by sexual motives. They are, however, directed towards a new goal—in particular artistic and intellectual activities, as Freud believed. The pleasurable absorption in intellectual challenges, learning, and intellectual exploration are a central focus in the latency period, as we will see in Chapter Two, section 2.1.1.

Freud borrowed the concept of sublimation from chemistry, where it describes a solid body changing directly into a gas under heat and then back into a solid but pure aggregate when cooled. A second connotation comes from poetic metaphor, where "sublime" motives—as opposed

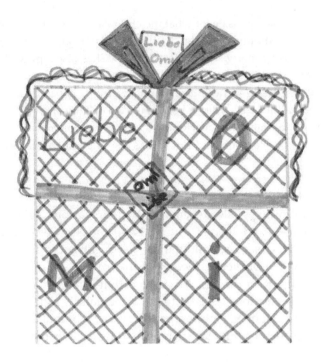

Illustration 7: Another drawing by Katharina: A Present Packed for Grandma.

to ridiculous or morally inferior ones—are attached to a work of art meant to be uplifting and approved by society. The word "sublime" is employed particularly with regard to fine arts, where it implies rarefied, inspired, subtle work. Accordingly, a culturally recognised activity that constitutes a "purified" or "sublime" form of the original sexual drive is called "sublimation". The capacity for sublimation is common in creative and artistic activity.

In her essay "Early Situations of Fear as Mirrored in Artistic Representation" (1929), Melanie Klein points out the significance of a child's early fears. As an example, she describes how Ruth first drew a picture of her mother with wrinkled skin, faded hair, a depressed facial expression. After this destructive wish to make her young, attractive mother old and ugly was interpreted for her, Ruth was able to draw a different picture, where her mother was pretty, commanding, full of energy, with a cream-coloured scarf around her shoulders:

> The wish to compensate for what the child has done to her mother in fantasy ... the portrait of the old, moribund woman would be the expression of primary, sadistic destructive wishes, also representing what the daughter feels she owes her mother ... Depicting her later in full possession of her powers and beauty ... is based in guilt feelings ... This fear, which I have found to be very significant for neurosis and inhibited development, can on the other hand promote ego development and constitutes a strong impetus for sublimations. (406ff.)

How is sublimation manifested in the age group we are here examining? Children invest steady energy in their various activities: they construct houses and towers out of Lego blocks, traverse complex ways with matchbox cars, build garages with entrances and exits; they make patterns out of blocks, piece together mosaics, draw pictures of meadows, animals, and cities. All these activities are eminently bound to real things—and to a lesser extent, to the child's inner desires and tensions. In this manner, children practise their motor skills and newly learned civilisation techniques such as reading and writing.

Interpretation

The flower, accompanied by a friendly sun, takes up the entire page. The artist—nine-year-old Katharina—shows us a harmonic structure in her work. She herself might be the flower that she has decorated with various colours. With its wave-shaped rays, the sun could represent Katharina's view of her mother or her parents' warmth and protection. The three butterflies presumably represent her friends, with whom she enjoys playing.

The second drawing shows a wrapped package intended for her beloved grandmother. It has a pattern and a green ribbon. The address shows us not only that Katharina can already write, but that she enjoys "playing" with the letters.

These joyful drawings should not divert us from acknowledging that in them, a wish is also expressed: the world ought to have such harmony. Behind this image, inner conflicts may be hidden—conflicts that remain in the background during this phase of life as long as good experiences predominate.

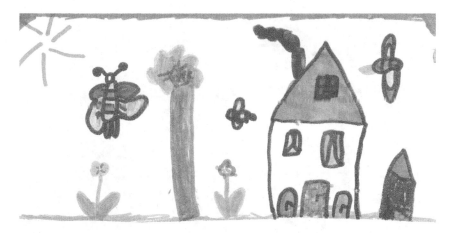

Illustration 8: Drawing by the six-year-old, Sebastian: House with Garden.

Interpretation

In his drawing of the house with its tree, lawn, flowers, and butterfly, Sebastian demonstrates how he has internalised a stable relationship to his maternal home. This house has three entrances, with the largest one presumably for the father and the two smaller ones for Sebastian and his older sister—all three of them have access to the mother's love. The smaller, tower-like structure could stand for him and his awareness that he is a small man who still has to grow. The large tree is on the other side of the house, and could represent his father.

In a picture of a submarine Sebastian drew somewhat earlier, stormy feelings come to the fore. The large submarine—indicating a strong self-image—fills the entire picture. From every porthole, massive amounts of steam emerge—in Sebastian, stormy feelings seem to be welling up to the surface. The butterflies are only sketched in lightly, as if creative and peaceful thoughts are not yet ripe. There is an anchor, but it has not reached the bottom. These drawings embody a form of reaction or sublimation: the child's emotional situation is expressed in artistic form.

Reaction formation

When we speak of the defence mechanism of reaction formation, we mean that unconscious defence mechanism tending in the *opposite*

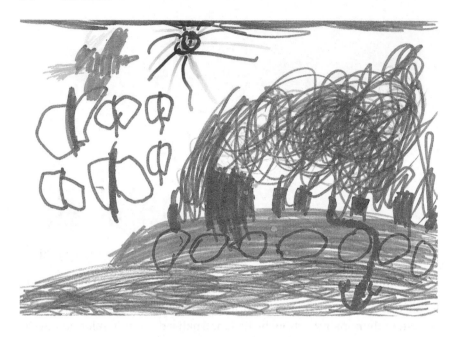

direction from the child's actual (suppressed) wish, hence, a reaction *against* it. For instance, the child's unconscious exhibitionistic wish to exhibit his naked body for admiration is reversed when he covers his body shamefully, perhaps also hiding from his parents while undressing. Reaction formation is unconscious, that is, the child exhibits shame and can find reasons for this, while remaining unconscious of his opposite wish lying behind this behaviour. For the parents, such a sudden reversal can be incomprehensible, and they ask themselves if they have not perhaps done something wrong towards their child. And yet this new, exaggerated sense of shame represents a station in the child's emotional development. Reaction formation is manifested in rigid, exaggerated behaviours—as well as in little slips revealing the child's hidden wish. For instance, a child attempting to hide her naked bottom might do this in such a clumsy manner that her entire body is now visible, and only her head covered. The exaggerated, almost parodic tenderness shown to a younger sibling can be an indication of murderous jealousy. It is helpful to understand and tolerate the child's split sexual or aggressive motivations. Parents who succeed in talking with their child about the feelings behind her behaviour will help her to find a way to meet the new demands of modesty or cleanliness. These sorts of reaction formation remain in later life as a conspicuous (although not to the person himself) cover for his true but unconscious affects or fantasies. The term "reaction formation" already indicates that it stands in direct opposition to the unconscious wish. Freud describes this intrapsychic process in the following way: first the wish is suppressed, and then stabilised through an anticathexis. In latency, such a process is normal, when cruel impulses lead to pity and wishes for chaos lead to conscientious reflection, or when the wish to besmirch leads to cleanliness. For compulsive neurotics, these opposing poles lead to an alteration in the ego. In the case of hysteria, the polar opposite is harder to detect:

> The conflict due to ambivalence, for instance, is resolved in hysteria by this means. The subject's hatred of a person whom he loves is kept down by an exaggerated amount of tenderness for him and apprehensiveness about him. (…) A hysterical woman, for instance, may be specially affectionate with her own children whom at bottom she hates; but she will not on that account be more loving in general than other women or even more affectionate to other children. (Freud, 1926d, p. 157)

Reaction formation in latency children is usually a transitional phenomenon, employed towards mastering the threat of sexual impulses and drive wishes. Parents and teachers can usually recognise this phenomenon through the child's extreme form of representation—for instance, exaggerated cleanliness corresponding to a repressed wish to play with body excretions; exaggerated embarrassment corresponding to blocked exhibitionism. Such exaggerated cleanliness tends to begin abruptly, accompanied by a disproportionate disgust for anything slimy or gelatinous. When the same child who enjoyed exhibiting her body, running naked through the house and laughing when getting dressed, now suddenly retreats into a corner shamefully or insists that everyone closes their eyes when she goes to the bathroom, the reaction formation and the underlying wish are easy to recognise. How can parents and teachers deal with such situations? Actually, it suffices to recognise and accept this development as a transitional phase. It is not always easy to keep a straight face, since such modesty or embarrassment appears comically touching in such a young person. However, when we can intuit the child's great fear of stormy repressed sexual desires in the background, such manifestations of reaction formation are easier to tolerate. Often, the behaviours of reaction formation facilitate a secret satisfaction of the suppressed impulse, for instance when genitals must be particularly thoroughly washed during a cleaning ritual or when the child's naked buttocks are visible through the blanket that should ostensibly hide them.

Denial

By the defence mechanism of denial, Freud means the refusal to recognise the reality of a traumatising or embarrassing observation. This constitutes neither deception nor a lie, where the liar asserts something she knows to be untrue. Rather, it is a deeply unconscious process unbeknown to the person—who speaks in all honesty: such knowledge simply does not exist. Freud employs this term to describe a phenomenon common to many of his patients in their childhood, who had no conscious knowledge of the anatomical difference between boys and girls. Freud traces this denial of an easily observed difference to the boy's attendant fear of losing his penis—which his father, whom he sees as a rival for the mother's love, will sever from his body. Freud called this fantasy rubric the castration complex.

In the phase of mid-childhood or latency here investigated, the energy of sexual impulses is diverted to other areas, whereby the control of body functions—toilet training, mobility—is already taken for granted. If there are relapses in this area, other children distance themselves from the relapser with scorn, or the "relapse" is collectively suppressed, as in the following example. Nobel-prizewinning author Alice Munro begins her short story "Pride" with the following sentences:

> Some people get everything wrong. How can I explain? I mean, there are those who can have everything against them (…) Make mistakes early on—dirty their pants in grade two, for instance—and then live out their lives in a town like ours where nothing is forgotten (…). (2012, p. 157)

Munro points out that even in later life, such an "accident" is employed to characterise a person. This pronounced reaction indicates the great significance that body control and the construction of a bulwark against early childhood carry. In the following case study (taken from a psychoanalytical observation of a working situation in the framework of the university course of study "Personality Development and Learning" in Klagenfurt), a child has wet his pants; in this case, the child is hardly an inferior student, but the head of the class, and not in some inconspicuous situation but in the middle of a lecture he was handling with ease. Thus, two opposing emotional currents clash: the star student gives an impressive lecture in as accomplished a fashion as the other students might aspire to; yet in the middle of the lecture, he wets his pants—something the other students all fear for themselves, potentially causing mirth or ridicule. How do the students, the class, and the teacher deal with this situation? The student's quick wit and the collective unconscious afford a creative solution—an example for the creative potential of the unconscious.

In her master's thesis, Maria-Theresia Strouhal (2014, pp. 38–57) describes the conflict situation in school:

> A ten-year-old student, whom Strouhal calls Ben, was assigned to give a report on billiards. Ben has a close relationship to his father, is self-confident, very intelligent, and loves "masculine" sports, including billiards. Frau Strouhal is the principal of this grammar school. When she meets Ben with his portable billiard table in the lift and learns of his planned report, she spontaneously decides to come and listen to it.

"In the nine o'clock break, Ben comes to my office and asks if I have the time now, he would like to begin with his report. I do indeed have time and accompany him to his classroom."

Ben demonstrates the ambitious wish to give his (he hopes) impressive report before the school head. He seems to have no fear of going up to her office and letting her know the report is about to begin. He is happy that she accompanies him, although his excitement is kept under wraps.

"Ben had placed the billiards table in front of the chalkboard, with small 'professional' cue cards on a chair behind it, meant to serve as prompts during his report. The other students sat on the seats around him as when they watched a film."

Ben has identified with his teacher; she always tries to provide the children with a professional model of presentation, furnished with various presentational techniques. He wishes to demonstrate to her, to the other students, but also to the headteacher of the school that he is familiar with these techniques. The initial impression is of Ben's great ambition: he wishes to give not only an adequate report, but an extraordinary one—he wants to shine. Ben's excitement is presumably heightened by the presence of the school principal.

"When I entered the classroom, I heard him say excitedly: 'She's really coming!' The children seem glad that I could find the time."

We see already how strongly the children have unconsciously identified with Ben; they empathise with the great importance he attributes to his report, since the school's head has found time to attend. A little of this excitement touches her.

"Ben goes behind the billiard table and begins his presentation with great energy. He speaks self-confidently of the sport's origins and name. He pushes his long hair back from his forehead now and again, occasionally turning around to glance at his cue cards ... 'The most important thing is posture!', he explains. He describes exactly how the feet should be positioned while striking the ball, demonstrating first with his left foot and then with his right foot; he bends over the table, demonstrating arm and body positions. This is accompanied by Ben's confident, clear description ... Ben takes the cue in his hand, explaining and demonstrating how to hold it, how to move the arm from the shoulder, all this in a confident and energetic tone of voice. He also explains how to write the word 'cue', although he spells it incorrectly ... nobody corrects him. Then he turns around once again and after glancing at his prompt cards, says: 'And now for the other thing we need: the balls!' He places two balls on the baize. He bends forward, putting his left hand on the deck and raising the cue with his right arm."

Ben's entire presentation radiates success; his descriptions and demonstrations are self-confident and skilful, and his audience of fellow students, teacher, and school head listen attentively. In her master's thesis, Frau Strouhal analyses the situation in considerable detail, hypothesising about Ben's inner reality.

Now, the moment of Ben's wetting his pants occurs. In the observation report, this is not mentioned, but in Strouhal's master's thesis it is described as follows:

> "Remarkably, this key event of Ben's wetting his pants is not mentioned in the observation report—only at the end, and indirectly. This is a clear sign that the observer was so strongly affected that even hours later, when she was writing the report, she could not

find words for what had happened. The absence of words can
signify the impossibility of reflecting on an event". (p. 46)

Both levels are interesting—why Ben at exactly this moment had
such an uncontrollable urge to urinate, and why the observer
could not put this event into words. But first, the events as they
occurred:

> "Suddenly, Ben stands up straight and exclaims: 'What's this?
> I've been sprayed with something!' He looks up to the ceiling and
> says: 'Is something dripping from up there? Is there water coming
> through?' His jeans show dark patches running on the inside of his
> thighs to his feet."

(Here, the author adds that in recent years there actually were
water leaks in the school, visible for instance in the hall outside this
classroom.)

The other children look in amazement at the ceiling, and one says:
'Yes, it's dripping from up there!' There is a small puddle on the floor.
The children start guessing where the water might come from, and take
the puddle as proof that it came from the ceiling …

"The teacher and I exchange glances, and I automatically take her
key ring from her desk as the teacher says to Ben: 'Come on, go along to
the bathroom and fix this …'"

(The school head accompanies Ben to change his pants—he changes
into sweat pants—and then returns with him.)

When he returns to the classroom, the children are again sitting in
their chairs, the teacher was perhaps speaking about the billiard balls'
momentum and different types of shot. At any rate, the children are
absorbed by the subject and are eager for Ben to continue with his
report and demonstrations. As before, he speaks in a lapidary fashion,
obviously enthusiastic about the sport … often, he tries out different
shots, some successful, some not. When a shot is successful, Ben is
pleased, and the children applaud."

This phenomenon—that the students did not trust their own sensory
perceptions of Ben's wet trousers, the puddle on the ground, and the dry
ceiling, instead accepting his explanation—represents a collective denial
of reality. The children defend themselves against the embarrassment of
Ben's loss of control, identifying with him. The sensory perceptions are

blocked, since the unconscious wish to protect an admired fellow student from embarrassing reality is greater. Later, Ben even said in a reproachful manner: "I can't explain it. Maybe my pants were wet before?" (p. 50). Logical thought is derailed; the threatening content is altered so as to be acceptable. Ben is also able to continue his report and further shine. The children applaud at every successful shot. Even after they have left the class, they continue to accept Ben's explanation unquestioningly.

As a defence mechanism, denial does not signify a conflict between ego and id; it is a denial of reality itself, in this case through the wish not to subject Ben to scorn and ridicule. Freud writes:

> The poor ego (…) serves three severe masters and does what it can to bring their claims and demands into harmony with one another (…) Its three tyrannical masters are the external world, the super-ego and the id. (1933a, p. 77)

Thinking supports the forming of compromises that allow drive desires access to consciousness, where the laws of logic and causality are operative. The logic of such a compromise is: I got wet, since the ceiling is dripping, just as it was the other time when there was water damage. The threatening content—the fact that an admired fellow student has wet himself—can be modified, so that it poses no threat to the boy's self-respect.

We can see the pants-wetting itself as an expression of Ben's tense, driven ambition. Freud (1905d) contends that every intense affective process can affix itself to the child's sexuality. A tension during the accomplishment of a difficult task can be manifested in genital excitement. In his *The Interpretation of Dreams* (1900a, p. 225), Freud points to the link between ambition and bed-wetting as a character trait.

The examples of blocked affect described here demonstrate how closely psychosexual and emotional dimensions are linked.

Psychosexual development

Even in this relatively calm phase of drive development, there can still be outbreaks of sexual desires and fears. Freud writes: "From time to time a fragmentary manifestation of sexuality which has evaded sublimation may break through; or some sexual activity may persist through the whole duration of the latency period until the sexual impulse emerges with greater intensity at puberty" (1905d, p. 178). In

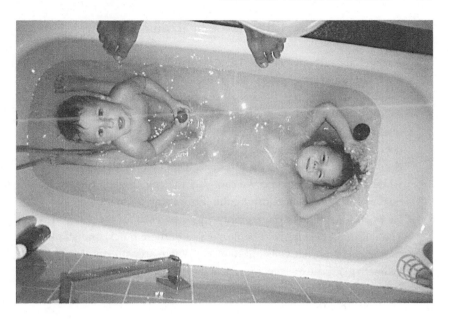

her book *The Psychology of the Woman* (1948), Helene Deutsch notes that sexual urges do not wholly vanish. "Upbringing strengthens the ego in its struggle for liberation from infantile drives and helps it to adapt to reality and the environment … tenderness should supplant drive needs, activity should supplant infantile aggressions, etc." (p. 8). Even if the infantile sexual impetus is now primarily directed towards other goals, it informs these other activities—as in sexually charged jokes, or when songs of rivalry are sung during play with a skipping rope.

The mastering of these suddenly erupting sexual urges and desires is channelled into games or jokes—as analysed by Erika Clowes (1996) in the Anglo-Saxon joke of the "farmer's daughter", a case of mastering Oedipal themes. Clowes distinguishes between two aspects of the joke's point: 1) the Oedipal triumph, and 2) castration fear. Within the framework of the joke, its narrator can work out his fears in relative security, his energy diverted to the listeners' laughter. The theme of separation from the family, suppressed during latency, the insecurity of sexual identity, and the revival of incestuous desires—all of these themes are addressed in jokes. Through joke-telling, social taboos and socially desired behaviour become anchored. Forbidden themes are addressed in the joke and suddenly defused, since a link to unconscious sexual wishes is established. Here are two examples of this.

The first joke is connected to the Oedipal triumph:

> A travelling salesman stopped at a farm and asked for a room for the night. The farmer says OK, but the only bed is with his young beautiful daughter. He's heard all about these travelling salesmen, so he puts up a wall of eggs between the two, and warns the salesman not to come near his daughter. During the night the salesman gets horny, and goes to make love to the girl. Of course he breaks the eggs crossing the bed, but the girl says, "Don't worry, I've got some white Will-Hold glue, and we can glue the eggs together again." So they did, but in the morning the farmer wants scrambled eggs. He breaks a couple of those empty eggs and goes for his shotgun. The salesman decides he'd better get out of there quick, and starts running. The farmer yells out to him, "Where are you running to? I want to get those roosters for wearing rubbers" (Folklore Archives, Jeffrey Landres; quoted in Clowes, 1996, p. 438. See also Burrison, 1989, pp. 186–187)

From the outset, it is clear that the narrator (and the listener) is identified with the clever travelling salesman. In his fantasy, the travelling salesman returns to his family after separation. This theme of the fatherless child is a typical motif in latency literature, describing the incipient detachment from the parents. The return to the family is often motivated by external conditions—a storm or the onset of night. In this way, early Oedipal desires for the mother, or redirected to the sister (who lives alone with the father), are activated. The father fulfils the salesman's wish only under the condition that he agrees to the prohibition of sex. This prohibition stands for the incest taboo, but also for the child's stringent superego. The main theme here is the father–son relationship. In this joke, the boy triumphs over the father, who is also too stupid to catch him. When the farmer sees that his eggs are empty, he believes the cocks are impotent. The father can no longer control his family's sexual behaviour, and the travelling salesman/son triumphs over him.

The second joke is linked to castration fears:

> Having been stranded by a broken-down car, the travelling salesman asks to stay in the farmer's house. "Only if you don't fuck my daughter," he is told. "Okay, you can trust me," he tells the farmer. Late that night the farmer's beautiful daughter slips into the salesman's

bed for a heavy session. But she falls asleep with him and the farmer discovers them in bed together in the morning. At gunpoint, he takes the salesman to the barn. The farmer takes the salesman's cock and puts it in a vice. He then tightens the vice down all the way before breaking off the handle. As he pulls out a large knife, the salesman stammers, "You're not really going to cut it off are you?" "No, you are," the farmer replies; "I'm just going to set the barn on fire." (Folklore Archives, Kenneth Schneider; in Clowes, 1996, pp. 442–443)

This second type of joke has more of a masochistic flavour. The child is meant to punish himself for his incestuous thoughts and desires. This joke aims to solidify castration fears: it is better to relinquish forbidden incestuous desires. The farmer's touching of the salesman's penis (standing for the penis of the boy telling the joke) also supplies a homoerotic element, and the farmer's gun is big and fearsome just as the father's penis is. Here, we see a symbolic domination through the father's authority. The strong anal/sadistic elements are typical for the latency child.

These jokes are told exclusively by boys and make for great amusement; forbidden words can and indeed must be spoken. Telling such a joke reduces sexual tension within a peer group, thus fostering emotional development and conveying emotional stability through verbal wit in a socially acceptable fashion.

With girls in latency, masochistic fantasies of being beaten often occur. Indeed, Clowes (1996) believes that childhood masturbation does not decrease in latency from early childhood. In his essay "A Child is Being Beaten", Freud wrote of one girl's daydreams, where she became sexually aroused imagining herself as the spectator of a scene in which a child was beaten. In such daydreams, the child beaten is usually the daydreamer's younger sibling. Freud understands the affective connotation of this fantasy in the first phase as follows: "My father is beating the child *whom I hate*," and, as the fantasy proceeds: "My father does not love this other child, *he only loves me*" (1919e, p. 185, italics in original). In a second phase, Freud sees the content of the daydreams, which leads to compulsive masturbation, as: "I am being beaten by my father." Access to these fantasies results only from further analysis. The blows represent a fantasised punishment for incestuous desires. This desire for coitus is replaced by blows to the buttocks. In these daydreams is hidden a pleasure elicited through pain, which we understand as masochistic pleasure. Freud writes: "This being beaten is now a convergence of the sense of guilt and sexual love. *It is not only the punishment for the forbidden genital relation, but also the regressive substitute for that relation*" (ibid., p. 189, italics in original).

In the third phase of this fantasy, a stand-in (usually a teacher) is beating another child. The daydreamer is a voyeuristic observer of a sadistic scene. This constitutes a regression to the anal-sadistic stage of sexual development. The fantasy is a means to strong, unequivocally sexual arousal and is employed as stimulation during masturbation. This childish perversion can be the foundation for a perversion persisting through the person's entire life, or it can be broken off, remaining in the background of a normal sexual development.

Another outlet for sexually coloured behaviours is jumping in a rubber ring, most popular with girls in this age group and one often pursued for hours on end. During the jumping, phallic and anal/sadistic rhymes are sung (Goldings, 1974).

A troublesome little brother is drowned in rhyme while the girls jump:

> I had a little brother
> His name was Tiny Tim
> I put him in the washtub
> To teach him how to swim
> He drank up all the water
> Ate up all the soap
> He died last night
> With a bubble in his throat.
> Fudge, fudge call the judge
> Mamma's got a newborn baby
> Ain't no girl, ain't no boy,
> Just a plain old baby.
> Wrap it up in toilet paper
> Put it in the elevator.
> First floor—miss.
> Second floor—miss.
> Third floor—miss.
> Fourth floor—KICK IT OUT THE DOOR.

(Goldings, 1974, p. 438)

These rhymes accompany the girls as they take turns jumping with the rubber ring, and afford a cathartic reaction of forbidden aggressive and homicidal feelings of jealousy towards the little brother. Interestingly, such rhymes are always about younger brothers, never younger sisters.

Girls form intimate friendships—where, however, a third girl is excluded (in fact, often several in succession) and to whom unflattering aspects of the first girl's personality are attributed: "She always has to win!", "She always wants to be in the centre of things!", "She steals your friends", etc. These behaviours undoubtedly result from the stringent superego of latency, with attendant guilt feelings, and occur only in girls (see Mertens, 1996, p. 127).

Sexual abuse and the failure to speak of it

Only in the last ten years have a multitude of accusations been made against teachers, caregivers, and priests who have sexually abused children between six and eleven years of age. Unlike the case of other bodily injuries in early childhood, parents or other authorities are surprisingly seldom informed of these cases of abuse, although children of this age can already express themselves fluently. Often, forty years pass before such traumatic experiences are discussed. The following two situations are described by way of example:

Example A

In his memoirs, *Little Did I Know. Excerpts from Memory* (2010), Stanley Cavell, a renowned philosopher and Harvard university professor, describes how he was sexually abused by his piano teacher as he played piano. Cavell begins by remarking that he never told his mother why he stopped playing piano. Then he describes his piano teacher, who walked with crutches.

> He sat beside me on the bench. I had got well into my piece (the Mozart d minor piano concerto) when he reached under my arms and unerringly, through my pants, squeezed my penis, whose nervous erection (which I think I was until then not conscious of) evidently made itself obvious despite my clothes. He asked: "What have I got?" I neither answered nor moved. My memory is that we actually finished the lesson. I may have gone back two

or three times, or pretended to my parents to continue going, not being willing to tell them about this incident, or to think what it was I might tell them to warrant never going back to the lessons. But even ignoring my general lack of interest in what this teacher had to say about music, my new alarm and amazement at this man's mysterious life and intentions froze the situation. Whenever images of that episode have occurred to me, I have asked myself what an appropriate response to his advances might have been. What I remember feeling was not exactly fear, not exactly anger, not exactly guilt, not exactly pity. That there was a right to outrage did not occur to me. Perhaps this is an instance that prompts one to ask whether English lacks a word here. But where exactly is here? Is that the same question? Or have I answered that question? (p. 70)

Cavell's confusion is still evident after forty years—a confusion that made it impossible for him to inform his mother, a confusion over his own pleasurable, nervous reaction, his feelings of shame and fear, over the chill and incomprehension interrupting a child's life. The child is incapable of going for help, and remains alone with these overwhelming feelings. When the piano teacher calls up the parents, Cavell is surprised that they accept his explanation that he now wishes to play the clarinet instead.

There is a double burden involved: on the one hand the sexual advances, which often lead to sexual arousal without the child's conscious participation; on the other hand the perplexing sensation of arousing an adult, of altering him. Often the confusing feeling arises of power over this adult. With children who have an emotionally stable relationship to one of their parents, this feeling of power will be dominated by disgust, and they succeed in withdrawing from the relationship. If, however, they are emotionally neglected or feel isolated, there is a danger that they permit this kind of perverse closeness, although suffering under it. Alongside the traumatic experience of an adult violating a child's boundaries, a central problem is the attendant psychic confusion and the loss of trust in adults.

Example B

In his article in *The Guardian Weekly*, "The Abusers Could Still Be Teaching", Alex Renton describes the boarding school syndrome from the perspective of a "survivor group" ("Now boarding school has a symptomology 'survivor's group'") (2014, 27ff.). Renton first discusses the cruel punitive ritual of cane beatings, employed above all against homesick, tearful young boys. Instead of support from fellow students, brute force has the upper hand under the guise of order. Alex does not dare to cry, although he is plagued with homesickness. "If you wept out loud, the 10-year-old dormitory captain and his deputy threatened to whip you with a belt … they told us on the first night." With grim humour, the survivors attempt to deal with this situation. In sixty-two private schools, teachers have been found guilty of sexual abuse within the last twenty years. Renton describes a bizarre sexualisation of the entire boarding school environment, a system of rewards and discipline where sexual contact is compulsory and then rewarded. He recalls in the article:

> Lost in this warren is the classroom where, one afternoon when I was nine or 10, a hated and violent young teacher I will call Mr. X slipped his hand into my corduroy shorts and tugged at my penis. This was a known hazard—in return Mr. X gave you a Rowntree's fruit gum. Mine was a green one, nobody's favourite. Is this a memory I can trust? No doubt. I can feel my face against the rough tweed of his jacket, scratchy.

This memory still has a tangible quality for the narrator, but he can also hardly keep from doubting it: can it really be that something occurred contradicting the child's right to protection from adults, teachers, and educators? Boundaries are crossed and perverted in order to give pleasure to the adult and damage the child. Renton was sure he never told his mother of these events. Only now, after he sent her an article on sexual abuse in English boarding schools, did she answer and tell him he had in fact told of Mr. X. She immediately went to the school headteacher's wife to report this wrongdoing. Only now, after she reminds him of this, can he weep and put himself once again in the situation of a small, helpless schoolboy. Only now does he understand why teacher X soon disappeared from the school, after being called a traitor by the school head and especially cruelly punished. He reads the prize-winning essay he wrote back then. It is the simple story of a self-centred young boy who received a rabbit for his birthday. The story goes on to tell of the boy, careless and cruel, neglecting to clean the rabbit's cage and to feed the rabbit. His mother warns him to take better care of the rabbit. He punishes the rabbit by throwing mud and stones at him. When it finally dies, the boy cries while burying it. And yet when after some days a fox digs up the rabbit's body, the boy does not notice this. The last sentence reads: "Even the flowers on his grave were not renewed."

The author is reproaching himself for becoming such a selfish boy— he was broken as a person in order to become a useful citizen. From the psychoanalytic perspective, we understand this essay as a cry for help from a small, neglected boy. He is not being fed on the emotional level; nobody is taking care of him, with the result that something in him dies. But not even this is noticed. The greatest cruelty is to send him back to this school, where he is brutally beaten and sexually abused. But it is exactly this phenomenon that makes sexual abuse so traumatic; the child feels responsible for the abuse. Victim and perpetrator are ntimately bound to one another—with therapeutic help required to free the victim from his confusion. (The psychoanalytic understanding of sexual abuse and its consequences is described more fully in my book *The Early Years of Life* (2013).)

Dealing with Oedipal hemes

Now, we see an example of how a child's viewing of a film can over-whelm his psyche with aspects of the Oedipal configuration (jealousy, death of the father, rivalry, and guilt feelings). In order to understand a child, it is important to pay attention to the specific ways she deals with inner conflicts. Joyful laughing while watching a film indicates a cathartic identification. Intense weeping indicates an overwhelming affect that the child cannot process. The physical and emotional prox-imity of an adult and his or her participation, with discussion of the film, can help the child to sort out these conflicts and diminish fear.

Here, two children view the Walt Disney film *The Lion King*. First, a précis of the film:

> In the awesome African steppe is the "holy land", ruled by Mufasa, the mighty lion king. The film begins with the birth of his heir, lit-tle Simba. But his devious uncle Scar manipulates Simba into dis-regarding the law, thus endangering his life. Little Simba follows the whispered exhortations of his envious uncle, who represents his inner negative impulses. His father manages to save Simba from

danger the first time, but the second time dies. Plagued by self-reproach and guilt feelings, Simba flees. Luckily, he ends up with the cheeky Timon and the warthog Pumbaa, who provide him with good cheer and their motto "Hakuna Matata", introducing him to a hedonistic existence. Only when he meets his childhood friend, the lioness Nala, does Simba learn from her that his uncle Scar has assumed rule over the kingdom, and that the animals are threatened with starvation. With help from the monkey Rafiki, he recognises his responsibility to return and to accept the task his father intended for him. He battles against Scar and the devious hyenas. Simba admits his mistakes—but Scar, not he, is the murderer of his father.

The seven-year-old Katharina and the almost five-year-old Sebastian react to this film quite differently, in accordance with their respective stages of development. Young Sebastian at first did not want to watch the video because it always makes him so sad. His sister convinces him to watch it anyway, and their grandmother sits down with them. Sebastian sits on the grandmother's lap and his sister also cuddles up to her. When the lion father Mufasa dies, Sebastian emits a few sobs, and even his sister begins to cry. But when the funny warthog appears, they both laugh again. When Simba leaves, both children's involvement is palpable.

When the children go home, Katharina climbs on all fours up the three floors to their apartment and says she is Simba. When their grandmother asks whether she is the little or the big Simba, she answers "the little one", and runs happily—as free as a lion cub—up to their apartment door. Sebastian walks up the stairs alone. Almost at the same time, their mother arrives home and greets Sebastian enthusiastically. He falls upon her, clinging to her like a baby, burying his head in her shoulder—as if it were the end of the world; he cannot even answer her when she asks what is bothering him. She then takes him on her arm and hip everywhere she goes as she puts food on the table, then bringing him to a quiet corner of the room where she speaks soothingly and strokes him.

When their father arrives home soon after this, he is first greeted enthusiastically by Katharina, and then looks for his son in order to greet him. He takes Sebastian in his arms. Sebastian is allowed to sit on his lap for the entire meal, and they both eat from the same plate. The more tenderly his father gives him pieces of food, the more Sebastian recuperates emotionally, then beginning to eat with gusto. He asks to be put to bed by his father and goes to sleep quickly. The next morning, he is again cheerful and jumps about with élan.

Katharina asks her grandmother to sit next to her. She shows her her homework, which she has done all by herself. Then she takes a schoolbook, reads the problems out loud, and requests her grandmother to watch her while she draws. When her father comes, she puts her pens away in order to run into the foyer and greet him.

Interpretation

Why do the two children react so differently to the film? How have they processed the film's themes, which actualise their inner latent conflicts?

Sebastian is in a transitory phase between the turbulent Oedipal phase and latency. This scene occurs three days before his fifth birthday; he is much occupied with the theme of growing up. He is counting the days until his birthday, since only then can he spend the night at his friend's house. He has an intimate relationship with his mother and an affectionate rivalry with his father, often leading to mock "fights". The film presumably actualised his Oedipal competition (the wish to kill his father in order to become the mighty king), and Sebastian is overwhelmed by guilt feelings, as if he himself had killed the mighty Mustafa (and his own father). He needs comforting from his mother, since he has regressed to an earlier stage of childish feeling and is afraid that his fantasies could become reality. He has to make sure that he is worth loving and that his father is not angry at him, indeed giving him food from his own plate—a step towards identification with the powerful father. At the same time, through this communion Sebastian can believe that he magically acquires his father's strength. Eating from the same plate seems to constitute reconciliation: now, his (inner) father is no longer angry at him.

The rivalry evoked by the film is something Sebastian has exhibited for the past few months. His father is able to deal with this in a playful way. For instance, when Sebastian manages through trickery to avoid his father's wish for him to change into a long-sleeved shirt from a short-sleeved one, the father is irritated. Sebastian then disappears, puts on his knight's suit, takes his play sword and assumes a fighting stance in front of his father. His father has to exert self-control to not laugh out loud; instead, he "stands his ground" in order not to contravene Sebastian's self-emancipatory gesture.

Sebastian's sister, two years older than he, either was not so disturbed by the film, or can deal with it better. At first she identifies with Simba, "the little one", as she says. Like a lion, she runs up the stairs to the third floor on all fours. Then she turns her attention to homework and shows her grandmother what she has learned up to now—thus gaining inner certainty that she is no longer a little baby. She is versatile and talented, and her grandmother is meant to give her attention and admire her. Here, Katharina sublimates her emotional turbulence, diverting it into the safe paths of writing and reading—which function as an assurance that she is now big and grown up, with the earlier rivalry with her parents a "bygone". She is already a school-girl, not a baby anymore.

How was it possible for the parents to so easily master Sebastian's emotional turbulence? Hans Zulliger (1970) has pointed to the "healing power of children's play", since the child represents her inner conflicts in play and can thus often work them out. Something similar is true for the way parents deal with children's expressions of inner turbulence. Sebastian's mother can see from his behaviour that he urgently needs her comforting presence, and she allows him to cling to her like a two year old while she cooks. Without knowing exactly why Sebastian is acting like a small child, she allows him to live out his wish of receiving special physical attention. As we see through the conclusion of this scene, these experiences resolve Sebastian's feelings of guilt and of competition with the lion father. Sebastian is now once again the little lion, and his powerful father allows him to sit on his lap and eat from his plate. Emotionally, this means for Sebastian that his father wishes him to become as big and strong as he is. This experience relieves the fear of his unconscious wishes and enables his loving feelings to become stronger.

A harsh rejection, with no comprehension of Sebastian's need to be treated like a baby, would presumably have led to an escalation. Perhaps Sebastian would have broken or spilled something in order to confirm he was bad and needed to be punished—something we call the "unconscious need to be punished". His parents would presumably have become angry and criticised him for being so naughty and ungrateful after a nice day at his grandmother's.

How close to the surface Oedipal desires and childish fantasies of omnipotence are—concealed under a six year old's skills—is shown by the following scenes.

Julia has been invited to her grandmother's with her mother, where a couple of very close friends, Hertie and Ludwig, have also been invited.

Even while the table was being set, Julia made her wish known to use just as big a plate and cutlery as the adults. She then indeed ate her chicken soup quickly all by herself and with very good manners. Before her grandmother went into the kitchen to prepare the main course, she set up a small table in the dining room and asked Julia if she might like to do a puzzle while she waited. Julia agreed, fetched without prompting a small stool and set about doing the puzzle. In a practised fashion, she emptied out the puzzle pieces from the box, first sorting the edge pieces and starting to fit them together. Her grandmother, who had not known Julia could already put puzzles together by herself, looked over twice and praised her careful industry. When the food was ready, Julia's mother called her over to the table. She was allowed to select a piece of the baked chicken, and picked a relatively large one. Among the baby carrots she found a particularly small one, took it and said: "This one is like me." Then she ate everything on her plate like the adults, and was allowed to return to her puzzle. When she had finished the puzzle, she was highly praised by everyone, and Hertie made the suggestion that they should celebrate the puzzle with the cake they had brought. "We could put a candle on the cake and light it," added Julia. Together with the grandmother, they prepared the cake and brought it in. Julia began a birthday song and everyone sang with her. Hertie sang: "Happy birthday to you … dear puzzle." When everyone laughed, Julia wanted to sing the song again, with everyone singing "dear puzzle". However, when she was the last to get her piece of cake (along with the grand-mother), she reverted to a little girl and wanted morosely to escape to her mother's lap. Ludwig, who received the first and biggest piece, offered Julia to exchange his piece with her, an offer she accepted happily. While continuing her play, she then sat alternately on his lap and on Hertie's. When the time came to go home, she wanted Ludwig to help her put on her boots, and clung to his neck. Falling asleep later, she asked her mother whether she could marry Ludwig when she was old enough.

Interpretation

On the one hand, six-year-old Julia is filled with the wish to be big, not using children's plates or cutlery, but adults'. Her skills and perseverance have also increased amazingly in the last six months: she manages to put the puzzle together by herself and eat by herself, deriving great satisfaction from this. The adults understand and share in her enthusiasm. Her abilities are celebrated playfully. During this celebration, however, concrete thinking seems to have taken the upper hand. It is almost as if the puzzle is not her accomplishment but has taken on its own life—a life given it by Julia, as its mother: indeed, the puzzle's first birthday is being celebrated, with Julia its creator and mother. This aspect is also operative when Julia continually sits on the lap of the only man present. He is allowed to help her, and ultimately she wishes to become his wife; in her fantasy, she has conquered him—not yet, but in the future. Here, a compromise between a sense of reality and wishful thinking has become possible. With the baby carrots, Julia can estimate her size realistically. She has trouble tolerating the rules of etiquette that leave her with the last piece of cake. She is hurt, and feels neglected. Her (logical) objection to her grandmother's explanation—that the hostess should serve herself last—is: "You're the hostess, not me!" A girl her age in kindergarten could perhaps accept her younger brother pushing ahead of her and say: "You can serve yourself first, I'm older and can wait!"

These scenes from everyday life show that behind seemingly simple theoretical descriptions, particularities of every child's life story and her situation are at work. The patterns of early childhood and the turbulent Oedipal constellation are only covered over, further exercising their influence during the apparent tranquillity of latency—to be reawakened to their full power in puberty, where they will be ordered into new structures.

Instruction in rules of conduct and table manners is not primarily an intellectual problem, but an emotional one. The point is usually that the child must set the satisfaction of his own needs aside and offer precedence to the guest. This is how civilisation attempts to avoid possible conflicts through rules of politeness and conduct, such as an ordered queue to avoid crowding and fighting. But logic is often on the children's side:

> As Sebastian greedily stuffed himself with food, holding the fork down low and his head close to the plate, his grandmother said: "Sebastian, you can eat so nicely when guests are here. Why are you doing it so fast now?" With a surprised expression, Sebastian

looked around and said with a deep tone of conviction: "But grandma, there aren't any guests here!"

He was correct in his observation, and yet was not truly in the right. The situation is funny because he took this rule of table manners literally, but it was meant to be generalised and internalised as a habit.

Mastering emotions

Beginning school

An essential feature of latency is the child's entry into school—a new organisation alongside the already known and trusted family. Belonging to the class as a student constitutes a variegated task of adaptation and adjustment—even when the child has already been in nursery school or kindergarten.

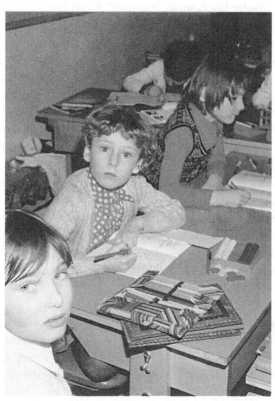

When starting school, the child leaves the world of early childhood and becomes part of a new system—the school, with its generalised rules, gratifications, and sanctions. He must find his place in this new world, left to his own devices for being accepted or rejected.

Psychoanalysis has shown that during important events, such as parting from the family or entering school, earlier experiences of endings are activated.

From its emotional significance, this new step forward can be compared with the first major alteration in the child's life: weaning. Weaning constitutes an important step towards gaining more independence. The baby can now ingest solid food, eat at the table with other family members, and be fed by persons other than her mother. The fashion in which the mother and her baby solve this task lays the foundation for transitions in later life. If the mother succeeds in introducing solid food carefully, weaning the baby slowly from the breast in a way he can accept, then the child can master partings later in life. If there was an abrupt end to breastfeeding, causing the child great pain and a feeling of abandonment, then entering school is also threatening and fraught with anxiety. Both transitions—weaning and entering school—constitute a large step in the direction of greater maturity and autonomy. Emotional transitions always signify parting, pain, and departure in the direction of something new. Feelings of grief and loss are set off by hope and joy—transitions are accompanied by mixed feelings. Schoolchildren often mourn for their earlier childhood. One child in therapy, who was hardly able to cope with the demands school made on her, openly expressed her longing for kindergarten: "Why can't I stay in kindergarten forever? I don't want to grow up, it's so hard." It was important to work through this pain and disappointment with her, to take her feelings seriously and not attempt to convince her otherwise.

School demands greater concentration, attention, and perseverance than kindergarten does. The class is larger than the playgroup in kindergarten. School buildings are bigger and harder to comprehend—it is not always easy to find the classroom. Children are afraid of getting lost. The new environment is confusing and often alarming, even though children are happy to go to school in order to belong to the older stratum.

There is no child for whom school is unimportant. The way a child masters his new tasks at school opens or closes chances for his entire life, since here the foundations of the child's attitudes towards learning begin. From birth on, the child has been learning and amassing new skills. At the beginning of school, the teacher usually treats the new pupils with affection, as a kind of mother figure. In cooperation with the parents, teachers attempt to ensure a good start. How can the child manage to view learning as a satisfying, goal-directed task, similar to putting together puzzles in kindergarten? How can this positive basic attitude be preserved in light of the undeniable fact that work is not only fun but also troublesome, requiring practice and patience? Even difficult assignments can be introduced in a playful way, and the child can receive appreciation for her determination and persistence.

Often, over-challenged schoolchildren revert to an infantile mode, wishing to be carried and bottle-fed. School's new and exciting experiences—often accompanied by a feeling of aloneness—usually are manifested in great physical fatigue at the end of the day. Some children show their fear and tension through sleeping disorders and morning headaches or bellyaches. A child in this situation longs for his parents' understanding and confidence that he can master this new development.

Belonging to this new system of relationships also entails a change in emotional priorities; instead of parents and caregivers, the teachers are the highest authority figures in this environment. The child trusts in them, they set and decide the demands made upon him. For parents, it is often painful to see their central position in the child's life modified.

At school or in the school building, a child sometimes projects her unconscious feelings if she herself is unwilling to recognise them when they are forbidden, embarrassing, or unpleasant. Here an example:

> One patient, Herr A., who had just had a second child—one he wanted, but whom he now sees as coming between him and his wife's body—told after a long summer vacation of when he began school: "I never wanted to go to school. My first day at school was terrible. The school building was huge, grey, and cold—like a monster I had to enter. I was scared and wanted to stay at home. I didn't even want to go to kindergarten."

Interpretation

When we discussed this sequence, it emerged that the patient wanted to possess the therapist completely for himself and viewed the summer vacation as a difficult interruption that only increased his hunger to be the sole object of her attention. This intense wish—his impulse to ingest the therapist in order not to have to share her with others ("I like you so much I could eat you up")—gave him guilt feelings. He was overwhelmed by this turbulent guilt and perceived himself as a monster. He projected these "monstrous" feelings, which he had also had as a boy for his mother—who was his sole parent the first four years of his life—onto the school and the school building. His experiencing of the school building as cold and grey was partly based on reality. Many older school buildings seek to emphasise the "seriousness of life" in contrast to playful kindergartens, and are built like barracks. Modern school buildings tend to fulfil children's wish for a colourful, cheerful environment where they feel at home. For the most part, however, the patient's "monster" image would seem to originate from his inner world: he was intimidated by his own monstrous greed and therefore could not consciously recognise it, instead repressing it.

Helping children during their transition to school is a serious task requiring close collaboration between parents and teachers. Children's reactions range widely, from those children who enjoy learning to those who only reveal their innate insecurity and fear of failure for the first time in the school environment.

In kindergarten, six-year-old Frida had already done written assignments with great pleasure and attentiveness. Now, her mother has prepared her for "real" school, and she is able to concentrate on her studies there successfully. Her father showed her the way to school, practising it with her several times and accompanying her the first day. Her mother, who was sceptical of this challenge to her little daughter, followed her secretly the first days until she was convinced Frida was capable of going it alone. At the parent-teacher conference, the teacher told them she wanted the parents to let the child do her homework alone, without their checking for mistakes: only then could she know what the children were truly capable of and where they had problems. Consequently, while Frida did her homework at her desk, Frida's mother would take up some handiwork, although sitting in Frida's room. Frida created fantastical ornamented edges for the letters she wrote. After lively sessions playing in the park, she often played school with her younger sister, taking the role of teacher.

In this example, the focus is not on doing homework *per se* but on learning to work alone. It is presumably also difficult for the mother to offer her older daughter this much space while remaining in the background.

Lisa Miller describes two children, Terry and Adrian, who have different problems in learning but are nevertheless motivated by an understanding teacher and integrated into the class.

Already in kindergarten at the age of four, Terry was unusually independent and apparently a strong boy; he imitated the imposing manner of his older brothers, with whom he hung out on the street. The kindergarten teacher told Terry's teacher that behind Terry the superman was concealed a fearful, vulnerable boy, who perceived himself in a dangerous world without protection. Accordingly, his teacher took care not to let Terry play the role of the ill-behaved, menacing schoolboy. She set clear limits for him, preventing him from taking things from the other children or hitting them. At the same time, she was open to his needful side, which had been inadequately satisfied when he was a baby, since his mother had been over-challenged. When Terry felt insecure, he was quick to become the superman. When his achievement in school worsened during his second year, he adopted the attitude of "I don't care". He began to steal, since his older brothers also did so. The school recognised his problems and supplied him with an advisory teacher, who was able to set him clear limits and demands but also gave him individual encouragement and support (see Miller, 1993, 34ff.).

Interpretation

The hiding of great vulnerability and neediness behind a hard shell or "cool" manner can lead to asocial behaviour and violence, when the hidden cry for help is not understood. Here, ignoring negative behaviour with a misconceived tolerance would be damaging, since every violent action evokes conscious or unconscious guilt feelings that are then blocked and compensated through obstreperous, arrogant behaviour. Children who have not been adequately held emotionally develop a kind of pseudo-strength—in order to hold themselves. Esther Bick (1986) talks of a "second skin" as manifested in an exaggeratedly muscular stance or a pseudo-intellectual attitude—as if the child could do everything for himself and does not need adults.

With children, stealing indicates inner problems, where they seek to fill an inner lack or emptiness. If the child received too little attention or love, he instead takes his mother's money, and things belonging to his siblings or his envied classmates. Stealing lends the thief a certain power: he can "purchase" attention through the stolen items. One girl told how she stole money from her mother to buy her a Madonna statue (the mother being particularly religious). Often, children buy sweets and chocolate with stolen money, either eating them or giving them to friends in order to obtain affection.

Adrian was an attractive, charming child; he was popular and enjoyed playing. In his first school year, he did not attract undue attention, although he only sometimes completed his schoolwork. In his second year, his new teacher observed Adrian closely and saw that behind his charming behaviour lay considerable insecurity. When she showed him his schoolwork was faulty, he at first smiled sweetly at her and tried to distract her; she then showed him what exactly his mistakes were, whereupon he became nervous, avoiding eye contact. One day he came home, collapsed in tears, and said he hated the new teacher and didn't want to go to school again.

Alarmed, his parents spoke with the teacher, who drew their attention to how Adrian avoided real learning—although in the two weeks before this talk his work had already improved. Adrian was convinced that he was not smart enough, and thus tried to get by with charm. This in turn served to cement his conviction that he was stupid and incapable—but that he could deceive adults, that nobody saw him as he truly was. The confrontation with his new teacher had already relieved his emotional burden, since he felt understood, albeit irritated by her. With his parents' support, he was able to work on his learning problem, since they encouraged him to do his homework, and practise his reading and maths even when the exercises were difficult and he didn't feel like it. Now he was able to achieve more, received praise, and began to believe in his capabilities (see Miller, 1993, 36ff.).

When the teacher confronted Adrian with his inadequate performance, this revealed his fear and was painful for him. However, in this case confrontation helped. He was able to improve his performance by working harder, with help from his parents.

Children in special education

When children have suffered deprivation in their first year of life, they are often unable to take part in normal classes and are taught in so-called "special" classes. Here are some scenes from observation of such a child, whom we call Max, from the thesis of Ulrike Wagner-Schick (2000):

Max is nine years old and has two half-siblings. Both fathers have been forbidden contact with their children. At weekends, Max is at his grandparents', although he does not like this since the grandfather is violent. Since he was a baby, Max (as well as his mother) has been physically abused by his father and his mother's many partners. His mother cares for him by taking him to one doctor after another, and is considering putting him in a psychiatric home. He has two fixed points in his weekly schedule: his Cub Scout group, which he loves, and psychotherapy, which he also likes.

Max's physical development is normal for his age; he is plump and has a round-cheeked face with large dark eyes. The group usually avoids Max—often he paces alone in the classroom. Tests indicate a delayed development of perceptive skills, as well as emotional and social deficits.

"When Max entered the special class in his second school year, he was strongly retarded and emotionally and socially at the level of a three to four year old," writes Wagner-Schick. In the early phase, his teacher was constantly holding him. She said: "Whenever possible, I took him in my arms. He drank from a plastic bottle lying in my arms and wrapped in a warm blanket" (ibid., p. 97).

As a baby, Max was deprived of the full quota of love, understanding, protection, and attention any baby should receive. Behind his uncontrolled behaviour, his great need becomes visible. He receives therapeutic help once a week, but his teacher also recognises that he is physically and psychically starved, and she finds a way to compensate for this.

Max is told to make longer words using the word "snow" (snowball, snow-fortress, etc.). He has great difficulty understanding this new task, especially reading the word "snow". He pronounces the first letter out loud, then calls for Ms R., since he does not know whether to put the second part of the word before or after "snow". First he reads "ballsnow" and shakes his head. Ms R. tells him to try it the other way around. "Max, what is a snow pile?" Max answers: "A pile of snow." He also knows that this noun is (in German) masculine. Then Ms R. tells him to write it down in his exercise book. Max writes the word, Ms R. stands behind him and strokes his head, then saying: "Yes, that's almost right," and pointing out the one letter Max misspelled. Max corrects his mistake.

Max at first does not know which order the words belong in. He does not emotionally know to whom he belongs—or who belongs to anyone. But in the special class, he has slowly learned to get help. It is important to him that the teacher stands in close proximity, providing him security. When he writes, she strokes his head gently as a mother strokes her baby. Step by step, Ms R. leads him to the correct solution. She lets Max show what he already knows and understands, thus fostering his self-confidence.

Once, Max is assigned a difficult subtraction. He needs his fingers for this. First, Ms R. helps him, and then he is asked to try it alone. He counts out loud, with Richard offering to help; he stands in front of Max and subtracts with him. Max calculates using Richard's fingers, and the subtraction is finished in no time. Max jumps up and rejoices: "Done, done, hurray! I did it, hurray!" Now he is allowed to have a break.

Through numerous small successes and a growing feeling of security and trust, Max begins to some degree to trust in himself. An empathetic fellow student can lend Max his fingers and thus become close to him. Max's joy at the successfully completed calculation is huge, and at the same time supplies impetus for further achievements.

Max's newfound self-confidence and the confidence of being able to perform calculations with help from his teacher and another student is the result of a long support process. In his first years at school, Max was unable to trust in his own achievements. When something failed or he broke some minor object, his self-loathing erupted. The following scene was observed:

> One time, Max pulled the top of his table off unintentionally, whereupon Ms R. took the table away. Now, Max began to chastise himself in the crudest language, crying and screaming. He seemed quite desperate. Ms R. came and held his right hand, speaking calmly with him while Max continued to berate himself. "Why am I so stupid?" he commiserated, hitting his head with his hand. When asked what he expected these blows to alter, he screamed desperately "Mommy, Mama …!" rubbing his tear-stained eyes and leaning his head on Ms R. (Wagner-Schick, 2000, 122ff.)

When Max breaks something, his whole world collapses. We presume that within him there is a stringent, implacable force that wishes to beat and berate him. Only the loving participation and calming words of Ms R. help him to find the way out of this cycle of self-castigation and self-punishment. In such moments he indeed hates himself, having so often experienced rejection from his mother and his father (who either does not take care of him or is not allowed to).

Close cooperation between the special education teacher and parents, as well as therapeutic help, are necessary to lay the foundation for emotional intelligence. Learning requires a capacity for bearing the psychic pain of not yet being able to do something. The teacher's aid is here essential, in order to give children confidence that they can learn. Unloved and rejected children can hardly develop the positive self-image and confidence for assimilating things new to them.

Psychoanalysis has always attempted to show that a modicum of emotional safety and love is necessary to learn and think. Especially with boys left by their fathers, the relationship to male teachers is important. Max has a close relationship to his teacher Mr. S.; here, physical contact is particularly important for Max, who has no contact with his biological father and has been rejected and beaten by his mother's partners.

When one of the two teachers is physically close to Max, he seems to feel himself accepted. Often, Mr. S. participates in a spat of fisticuffs with Max: "It's time now, it's time now," Max calls out and immediately runs over to Mr. S. This mock boxing match obviously gives Max pleasure, and he crows with delight. He boxes Mr. S.'s left arm, laughing and rolling his eyes. Mr. S. holds him tight, releases him, and Max allows himself to fall on the floor. He does this several times, chortling with pleasure. Max asks Mr. S.: "Will you hold me tight?"

Once again, we are reminded of the affectionate physical altercations between a father and son, as they wrestle, roll on the floor, or run after one another. The son can ascertain that his big, strong father touches him and "emotionally and mentally holds" (Winnicott, 1965) him without hurting him. In this game, love and rivalry can be integrated and expressed. Max's laughter shows how much he enjoys this. On a symbolic level, we can understand the playful grip and release as expressing convergence and separation—just as the teacher and Max separate every day and converge the next day.

Max challenges Mr. S. to afford him even closer body contact: "Now a nelson," he tells him, whereupon Mr. S. holds Max tight in a headlock. Max laughs and radiates joy. Then he grabs Mr. S.'s leg several times and lets himself fall.

Max enjoys his physical and emotional closeness to Mr. S.; perhaps he can demonstrate and work through his unconscious fear of a father figure in this game. Just as Max experiences loving closeness to his teacher, his psychotherapist, and bus driver, he can by the same token also comfort other students. He begins to develop the capability called "concern" by Winnicott (1963)—caring for another person.

Another student, Michael, has problems copying words from the blackboard ... Max springs up and goes back to Michael, saying: "Now I'll help you write it into your book." Max insists on reading Michael the exercises. He is sweet, his voice gentle, as he writes for Michael; this all happens very quietly ... Michael lies on the floor, with Max next to him. "Do you want to go to Ulli (their teacher)?" Max asks him. "I'll look in your schoolbag. There are nice things in there, anyhow ..." He discovers a photo and says to Michael: "Look, a photo. You look fine in it. You aren't really handicapped, you just think you are."

It is very important to Max to be the helper for once, not the helped. In this special class, this is made possible: the children are allowed to get up and offer help spontaneously—help which, in this case, Michael accepts. In the previous observation, it was vice versa: Michael loaned Max his finger to help him with his calculations. But Michael is now feeling sad, unable to keep working, and lies down on the floor. Max identifies with him and lies next to him, so that Michael is no longer alone. Evidently, Max is closely bound to Michael emotionally. He looks in Michael's schoolbag and finds a photo. At first he makes an affectionate comment as to how good Michael looks in the photo. Then he seems to become conscious of Michael's feeling of inferiority since he is in the special class. This question must touch Max as well, and his hopeful side tries to cheer Michael up, encouraging him to think he is not handicapped. We can see the contents of the schoolbag as a symbol for the contents of Michael's psyche.

From these observations, it becomes clear how important the emotional aspects of learning are: only when the child has someone emotionally involved with her on an intellectual level can the child take in learned content. Salzberger-Wittenberg, Henry-Williams, and Osborne (1997, 82ff.) write of a teacher's capacity for helping children to bear the psychic pain of ignorance, fear, and helplessness, in order that they learn from experience. Teachers in special education classes are particularly confronted by the challenge of helping children through their psychic pain and supporting them emotionally and mentally.

Changes in the emotional significance parents hold for the child

The new inner image of the parents—in early childhood elevated to mighty, idealised kings or queens, nourishing giants, powerful protectors—now begins to approach reality. The split-off bad side of parents, seen in the dangerous witch and sorcerer or the strict, vengeful god, is mostly repressed, as Melanie Klein (1946) emphasises. Parents are now not the only reality; the child becomes acquainted with other children's parents and other families and begins to doubt the incomparable and unique status of his own parents. Aside from these experiences from outer reality, there are inner dynamics of the child's new devaluation of his parents, pointed out by Freud in his essay "Family Romances" (1909c). Giving up the Oedipal desire for the opposite-sex parent is often linked to a sense of being set back; the child must share its parents' love with her siblings. The predominant feeling is that the child's loving tendencies towards her parents are not fully requited. Children may have fantasies that they are not truly their parents' child but instead a foundling or stepchild. One patient, her mother's favourite child, was told by her five siblings that the reason she occupied a privileged position was that she was actually a foundling: they pointed out that she had a different eye colour to her mother's or theirs, claiming that their mother was particularly nice to her only so that she would not realise that she was in fact an outsider. The girl soon believed this and did not trust herself to discuss the matter with her mother or father. It took psychoanalysis to discuss these fears and her guilt feelings at taking too much space in her mother's heart; these emotions then shed their threat for her, since now she could see them in relation to her jealous siblings' desire for revenge.

Daydreams, as a particular form of fantasy, often include the idea of being an adopted child or foundling. Fantasy is meant to fulfil wishes and correct reality. It pursues two goals, erotic and ambitious in character. Freud calls this phenomenon of fantasy the "family romance". He writes:

> At about the period I have mentioned, then, the child's imagination becomes engaged in the task of getting free from the parents of whom he now has a low opinion and of replacing them by others, who, as a rule, are of higher social standing. He will make use in this connection of any opportune coincidences from his actual experience, such as his becoming acquainted with the Lord of the

Manor or some landed proprietor if he lives in the country or with
some member of the aristocracy if he lives in town. Chance occur-
rences of this kind arouse the child's envy, which finds expression
in a phantasy in which both his parents are replaced by others of
better birth. (ibid., p. 238)

A second phase of the family romance comes into play when the child
acquires some knowledge of her parents' sexual relationship and
thus realises that her mother's identity is certain but her father's is
not. (This is expressed in the well-known legal saying "Pater sem-
per incertus est, mater certissima est".) Along with the knowledge
of the sexual act comes the tendency to imagine erotic relationships,
where the mother—as object of highest sexual desire—is fantasised
in situations of secret infidelity, thus supplying motives for revenge
and retribution. Often, the child imagines his mother with as many
illegitimate children as she has actual children. Freud: "… the hero
and author returns to legitimacy himself while his brothers and sisters are eliminated by being bastardized" (ibid., p. 238). Behind the
seemingly incorrigible cruelty of child fantasy are tender feelings that
are meant to be hidden and remain unconscious. Behind the child's
apparent disloyalty and thanklessness—since he wishes to replace a
loving father with imposing, new, and noble parents—the true character of his parents becomes visible. Freud understands this family
romance as "… the child's longing for the happy, vanished days … He
is turning away from the father whom he knows today to the father in
whom he believed in the earlier years of his childhood; and his phantasy is no more than the expression of a regret that those happy days
have gone" (p. 238).

Melanie Klein describes a latency child's altered relationship to his
parents as an alteration in psychic structure, where the child's mental
state is focused on working through and modifying early (paranoid-
schizoid) and mature (depressive) fears:

> When we observe them in the light of how fear develops, we can
> summarize the transformations characteristic of the latency period
> as follows: the relationship to the parents is marked by greater
> security; the introjected parents approach the image of the real
> parents; their standards and values, their admonishments and pro-
> hibitions are accepted and internalized, and thus Oedipal desires

can be more effectively suppressed. All this represents a peak in
superego development. (1952, p. 82)

Klein emphasises that the strengthened ego and superego can now
meet the demands of the real parents (objects) and the real world.
The precondition for a successful transition during latency is to master fears; this is founded in a positive connection of objects to loving,
restorative impulses towards parents, along with an improved distinguishing of reality (see Etchegoyen, 1993, p. 348). Hence, the child
becomes better adjusted to inner and outer reality, which leads to a
strengthened ego.

Behind the seemingly calm façade of latency as the golden period
of childhood, the "family romance" demonstrates the emotional struggle a child undergoes in order to emotionally distance herself from her
parents—a step forward that will later reach its turbulent peak in puberty.

Separation, loss, and death

Experiences of separation and the loss of loved ones are pivotal and painful in any period of life. Many adults believe they must shield children
from painful experiences and attempt to shield them from psychic pain,
neglecting to explain important matters or supplying the children with
lies and half-truths. However, this hardly constitutes protection, and
instead tends to make the situation worse—since fantasy explanations
for a person's sudden absence usually are far more painful than the true
explanation. Psychoanalysis holds that every child can bear the truth if
it is conveyed by a sympathetic person and the adult shares the attendant psychic pain with the child. Fantasy explanations for a sick adult's
altered behaviour or death can be far worse than the truth. Mourning
with the child and sharing his pain, on the other hand, brings child and
parent closer emotionally—which helps them both. A child's participation in a burial allows her to say farewell and to work through her grief
within the family framework, instead of remaining at home alone without the others.

Psychoanalysis devotes itself to the psychic working through of
these experiences. Freud, the great enlightener, was against the obscur-
ing of important life questions on birth and death, and understood
psychoanalysis as a process for approaching and understanding the
psychic truth of the self with its conscious and unconscious impulses

and motives. For Freud, sexual enlightenment is an essential moment for convincing the child of her parents' honesty. He spoke out against lies and half-explanations, and propounded an ongoing enlightenment of the child regarding sex and sexual differences (1907c). Wilfred Bion (1967) takes these thoughts further when he posits the concept of "ultimate truth", represented in the symbol "O". Truth is essential for intellectual development. According to Bion, the psychic apparatus cannot develop and will starve without truth. Analytical interpretations attempt to convey at least partial truths and lead to an integration, enabling psychic growth. According to Bion, the position of the analyst is comparable to that of a court jester, who offers risky truths in the form of jokes or from an ostensibly insane perspective, while uncovering unusual and bizarre configurations. Alongside the conscious wish of the analyst and patient to understand, we must also consider the unconscious disinclination to understand. Something in us blocks us against a painful or shameful truth.

One example of abrupt separation

In her memoir, *Home Is Everywhere*, Barbara Coudenhove-Kalergi describes how she experienced the completely surprising separation from her dearly loved nanny:

> At some point Rita left us. The adults agreed among themselves that we would not be informed. I was to be spared the traumatic farewell. No farewell, no tears. One day Rita was simply gone. She's at home in South Moravia, I heard: her family needs her. From Moravia, she wrote my mother letters and postcards with greetings to me. Mommy wants to read me these letters, but I don't want any part of it. I hold my ears shut and run from the room. I don't want to think of Rita, and don't want to be reminded of her—my Rita, who left me. It is too painful—a wound that never wants to be healed. This was the first true blow of fate in my life. (2013, p. 16)

Coudenhove-Kalergi describes a double wound: not only being deserted by Rita, but also not being afforded the chance to carry out a ritual of farewell—she feels she was not taken seriously. Without any forewarning, an intimate bond is broken by the sudden, secret departure of her nanny. The feeling of abandonment floods her, and she experiences this as a breach of trust, a betrayal. Beloved Rita becomes a rejected person: the child, irreconcilably insulted and traumatised, cannot and will not accept her greetings. Why do parents inflict this on their children? Their justification is to spare the child pain, but parents do not consider that because of their silence, it is impossible to deal gradually with the thought of inevitable separation. Perhaps Barbara's mother also was afraid to witness her pain at separation from the beloved nanny Rita— or perhaps she was jealous of this intimate bond.

The new nanny replacing Rita also is in a problematic situation: "At the age of seven, I certainly don't like her, especially since she isn't Rita" (ibid., p. 16).

Her negative feelings, disappointment, and the breach of trust were transferred to the new nanny, who has a difficult position—if indeed she has any chance at all of eliciting the child's trust. More likely, she will be confronted with suspicion; the child is now careful not to give somebody love and affection who will again abruptly disappear and leave her in the lurch.

Although it is now well known how unfavourably such sudden, unprepared separations influence children, switching teachers is often managed in this manner. The new teacher enters the children's life on the first day of school, and the children have to deal with her predecessor's absence; often, the new teacher has to begin her work with the openly or subliminally expressed recalcitrance of the children until she manages to build a new relationship.

For school as an institution, it is of great significance to prepare well a necessary switch in teaching personnel, allowing children insight into the reasons for the change such as pregnancy or the birth of a baby. A ritual of farewell is helpful. If it is possible to have the departing teacher introduce the new one and acquaint the children with her, then the children experience a continuum, as if they were being lovingly passed from one hand into another. The children's mixed feelings can then be discussed, in order to let positive experiences make the best of the transition. If the farewell can be well prepared, positive experiences and loving memories will retain their vitality (see Salzberger-Wittenberg, Henry-Williams, & Osborne, 1997, 178ff.).

The manner in which children deal with separation and farewell depends on their early experiences of separation. Birth constitutes the first experience of separation from the protection of the mother's body. Did the mother and baby succeed in cooperating on this venture? It is the baby who initiates the birth through his hormones, also stimulating the opening of the birth passage with his movements. The second separation is weaning—either from the breast or from the bottle—and the transition to solid food. Did the mother and baby succeed in managing a slow process of farewell, or was weaning an abrupt, unprepared event? Was the mother able to bear her and the baby's feelings and reflect upon them?

In the case of major illness or the death of a parent, too, it is fundamentally important to keep latency children involved. The intense fears and emotions of such times cannot be kept secret; children will intuit the situation. When adults attempt to conceal the truth, children also become unsure whether what they are observing corresponds to the real situation, and why parents seem to be misleading them.

The death of Benjamin's grandmother by a stroke—two days after celebrating her golden wedding—was a shock to the whole family. The ten-year-old grandson said in astonishment to the grandfather: "How can granny do this? She had such a lovely celebration and two days afterwards she pisses off? I am so angry with her." The grandfather answered from the depths of his soul: "You are totally right, Benjamin. I feel the same!"

Death embodies the ultimate form of abandonment, which also evokes a feeling of aloneness and irritation alongside grief. When children can discuss this explosive mixture of feelings and share them with an adult, it constitutes an important step towards integrating and working through them.

The capacity for feeling pain over the departure of a loved or important person requires that the child has built an emotional relationship with that person. Children who often have had to switch caregivers, if they have been taken from their parents and put in a home or given to foster parents, cannot develop such close relationships. They then search for closeness and contact to various persons in a fashion that can tax caregivers' capacities for maintaining contact. In the case of Max, already described above, Wagner-Schick made the following observations at her first visit:

> I had met Max already in the previous school year, when I was observing the special class. Back then, he was already eager for contact and not distracted by the three observers present. On

the contrary, I can remember that he came unusually close to us *strangers*, even cuddling with us. He seemed to have no feeling for appropriate distance. (2000, p. 98)

In this description, the contradictory feelings evoked in visitors by a new child's surprising behaviour emerge. First, Max is deemed "eager for contact", since he comes so close to the observers and cuddles with them. Only in the next sentence does an unpleasant tone arise, when the observer writes of "no feeling for appropriate distance". In fact, such children are capable of evoking in us the feeling that we are false, as if we promise them something we then do not supply.

This observer's reaction is surprising when she later returns to the class after seven months.

"Max comes over to me and recognises me again. He asks what I am doing here. I answer that I am here to speak with Ms R. and will return in two weeks … 'Are you a secret agent?' he asks. I deny this. 'No, she is from the police. She's looking the children over, whether they should be sent to a home,' says Max."

In my interpretation, I described Max's behaviour as typical for a neglected child, fabricating pseudo-closeness since he is unable to experience a true bond. Seven months later, this child—who has massive learning problems—not only remembers the person, but also shows he can clearly relate to people. What Max then says reflects his great fear of being sent to a home. In actual fact, his mother was considering putting him in a home. Very carefully, he approaches the observer and questions her specifically; however, he shows his mistrust and recognition that adults do not always show their true motives.

At a later point, Max shows grief over the loss of a loved person—in that he can express his wish that a person to whom he has built up trust should not leave the class:

"Max is used to going to school on a special bus for handicapped students. One day at school, he is sitting at his desk calmly and looking seriously around the classroom. Suddenly, he begins to weep. When Ms R. notices this, she comes to him, puts her arm comfortingly on his shoulder and asks him quietly what is the matter. Max continues to weep, but begins haltingly to explain: he is sad because the bus driver who brings them to school is no longer there. Today, there was another bus driver. But Max would

rather travel with the driver he knows, who was always so nice
and funny."

Max is in a special class, where his teacher Ms R. can precisely observe
him and help him to show his grief and discuss the reasons for it. The
fact that Max can only laugh with his usual bus driver and is sad when
he loses him illuminates the quality of his relationships in general. The
new driver may make him afraid.

"Max asks Mr. C. (the substitute teacher, whom Max has grown to
like) whether he has already looked at his homework. 'What did you
say about my designs, the stars and little crosses?' Mr. C. says they were
great … As proof of his affection, Max did particularly nice homework
and as a special present, has drawn ornamental letters in the margin"
(ibid., p. 101).

Affection for his teacher motivates Max to a special achievement.
The margin designs—for other children an expression of pleasure in
learning—express his successful relationship to Mr. C. At the farewell
party, Max can express his feelings and wish directly, saying: "I don't
want you to leave" (ibid., p. 102). He shows that he does not want to
lose the teacher. Max can show his love symbolically through his ornamental letters—and it is to be hoped that he can continue this after the
teacher leaves.

CHAPTER TWO

Latency: the development of thinking and learning

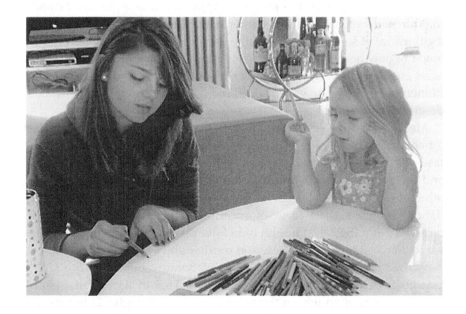

The forms of egocentric thinking characteristic of children—accompanied by fantasies of omnipotence and magical thinking—lose some of their importance during latency; so does the small child's mental occupation with her and her parents' body functions. The world beyond parents and family becomes interesting. The child's capacity for abstract thought increases. Suddenly, intellectual activities take flight. School capitalises on this new activity. An intensely curious child poses questions of his environment, particularly the questions of "why". Pleasure in learning gains the upper hand. Teachers and other educators find children highly motivated to learn and discover new terrain.

The biological basis for this development lies in a neuro-anatomical differentiation of the brain, a topic that will not be discussed in detail here. But which models of intrapsychic development does psychoanalysis employ towards understanding these developmental steps? Here, I will provide a short description of the theory of thought processes and learning as viewed in psychoanalysis.

Sigmund Freud examined thought processes in the unconscious and conscious areas of the psychic apparatus, thus radically extending our understanding. On the other hand, Freud also emphasised the significance of sexual curiosity in the drive for knowledge. Freud examined not only how thought first originates, but also which psychic processes enable symbolisation and the acquisition of language, doing so in numerous writings; however, space considerations preclude a detailed description here.

Melanie Klein takes up the concept of sexual curiosity as an impetus for acquiring knowledge, especially as illuminated by early archaic fantasies of aggressive penetration and examination of the mother's body and the child's interest in his own body—an interest later extended to other objects. Klein's concept of projective identification offers a foundation for the earliest form of communication—a form she herself believed pathological, although Bion later posited it as a general, incipient form of understanding between mother and baby.

Wilfred Bion (1967) developed an elaborate "theory of thinking" that links psychoanalysis with philosophy. This includes three parts: 1) the concept of an inborn "preconception" of thought, 2) the model of "container and contained", and 3) "learning from experience" as constituting an emotional experience aimed towards self-acquaintance, acquaintance with others and with the world; he dubs this rubric "K", for "knowledge".

I will also here describe Jean Piaget's developmental model for the building of cognitive structures and thought operations in latency children.

Freud's theory of development

The crucial characteristic of Freud's revolutionary view on the psyche is how he extended our understanding of consciousness through the unconscious dimension. Human thought processes are seen as one unity; the higher functions of reason—what Freud called "secondary process"—cannot function separately from primitive and archaic areas, called "primary process". In classical Freudian terms, the psyche is described metaphorically as a three-part space where the lowest level is the unconscious, the middle level the preconscious, and the uppermost level consciousness. He compares these layers to the spatial ratio between the invisible and visible portions of an iceberg, where 80 per cent (unconsciousness and preconsciousness) is under water, and only 20 per cent (consciousness) is above water. Psychic life thus occurs mostly at the unconscious level; psychoanalysis is the psychology of the unconscious.

Freud proceeds from a model of conflict between the psychic entities id, ego, and superego. In distinguishing between the systems of the unconscious, preconscious, and conscious, Freud observed psychic processes from a new point of view—depending on which "locations" in the psychic apparatus constitute the theatre for conflicts, or what entities are the stuff of conflicts. Desires, memories, and impulses that a person is unwilling to recognise are relocated into the unconscious, with a tendency to re-emerge later. In the system of the unconscious, there is no cathexis, the pleasure principle predominates, and the extreme facility of the unconscious in connotation makes for much conflation and (mis)attribution. Freud's "secondary process" may be established only later in life, yet it is present implicitly from the beginning. Thinking in the secondary process is rational, includes negation, an understanding of time, contradiction, with the reality principle predominating. "According to current research, secondary-process principles of organization completely assume the categorizing of conscious and unconscious psychic events from the seventh year of life onwards," write Brakel, Shevrin, and Villa (2002, quoted in Bohleber, 2013, p. 809). The dominance of primary process thinking, however, remains in effect for a person's entire life, even when drive desires and impulses are censored and diverted to higher goals.

As proof of the existence of the unconscious, Freud supplies in *The Psychopathology of Everyday Life*—one of his most popular writings—the "parapraxis" or Freudian slip, comprising a wide spectrum of seemingly insignificant phenomena such as forgetting or misplacing something, speaking incorrectly, and inappropriate gestures within normal behaviour. One of his illustrations was: the *Freie Wiener Presse* reported how the president of the Austrian Parliament, instead of declaring a session to be opened, declared it to be closed. As Freud interprets this: "His attention was only drawn by the general merriment and he corrected his mistake. In this particular case the explanation was no doubt that the President secretly *wished* that he was already in a position to close the sitting, from which little good was to be expected" (1901b, p. 58). The spectators' spontaneous laughter is a reaction to a communication from the speaker's unconscious, where tension is dissolved—a tension that cannot be consciously controlled. In the Freudian slip, the unconscious wish is fulfilled behind reason's back, so to speak, thrusting itself forward into manifest speech and thus successfully completing its mission.

Step by step through the beginning of adulthood, orientation towards the pleasure principle is replaced by the reality principle. Of this graduation, Freud observed: "Since the later care of children is modelled on the care of infants, the dominance of the pleasure principle can really come to an end only when a child has achieved complete psychical detachment from its parents" (1911b, p. 219). With the onset of the reality principle, however, "… one species of thought-activity was split off; it was kept free from reality-testing and remained subordinated to the pleasure principle alone. This activity is *phantasyzing*, which begins already in children's play, and later, continued as *day-dreaming*, abandons dependence on real objects" (ibid., p. 221). The period between six and twelve poses great demands on the child for how she deals with the reality principle. She must subject herself to the same demands, rules, and prohibitions as her larger peer group.

One question frequently posed by readers is: which behaviours are normal and which are pathological or problematic? Freud's answer to this question is rooted in his desire to understand neurotic thinking; consequently, he seeks to explain both normal *and* pathological psychic phenomena. "We no longer think that health and illness, normal and neurotic people, are to be sharply distinguished from each other, and that neurotic traits must necessarily be taken as proofs of a general inferiority" (1910c, p. 130). This is also the reason I introduce examples of child behaviour from "the spectrum of normality" here, to demonstrate how analysis helps work through (normal!) fears and inner conflicts in order to facilitate further development. Disturbing inner conflicts that are only later observed by parents can also be hidden behind innocuous behaviour. Generally, latency is a period where a child's positive learning habits and interest in the world should help him fulfil scholastic demands; most children enter therapy because they fail to match these expectations, due to inner conflicts that no longer can be suppressed. Deciding whether a child's behaviour requires therapy entails careful examination, as described later in Chapter Three.

Sexual curiosity as thirst for knowledge

In his *Leonardo da Vinci and a Memory of His Childhood* (1910c), Freud asks where the energy feeding Leonardo's passionate quest for insight originated. His answer was that this thirst for knowledge originates in the sexual curiosity that we can observe in small children. Children exhibit interest in their bodies and their parents' bodies. They attempt to discern anatomical sexual differences and want to know where they came from. They ask themselves what their father and mother had to do with their birth, how they came out of their mother's belly, and how a baby gets in there. Children develop various theories of sex, of birth, and of fertilisation, corresponding to their respective developmental phase: oral explanations—babies come from kissing or eating; anal theories—babies come from faeces or are pressed out from the mother's anus. Ideally, adults will answer children's numerous questions openly and in a manner appropriate to children, so that their quest for sexual knowledge is satisfied and they can proceed to other objects of curiosity. Freud calls this psychic mechanism of diverting curiosity and sexual energy to other (non-sexual) objects "sublimation" (see Chapter One, section 1.2.2). A child's later mental efforts towards solving intellectual tasks are based in a relatively stable sense of self; here, she must employ reason without allowing herself to be limited by authoritarian mental prohibitions and taboos. Freud believed this capacity for autonomous thinking and investigation plays a role not only in individual life, but has led intellectual history to an important phase of enlightenment and liberation of thought. Only since the Enlightenment did scientists such as Copernicus, Galileo, and Darwin dare to challenge the mental prohibitions of the Church, which for centuries dogmatically propounded that the world was the centre of the universe, was flat, and was created in seven days by God. Freud quotes Mereschkowski, the first modern scientific researcher, in the *Codex Atlanticus*: "He who appeals to authority when there is a difference of opinion works with his memory rather than with his reason" (ibid., p. 122). A capacity to rebel against the father is one precondition for this valorous attitude; another is the trust in one's own judgment. Freud describes the inner psychic preconditions for an "education towards independence", where the subject achieves autonomic thinking—which also entails experimentation and the testing of reality.

If the child's sexual questions are left unanswered, with the child branded as stupid or impudent, Freud believes there are three possible ways to react psychically: the first possibility Freud calls the "neurotic inhibition":

> Thenceforward curiosity remains inhibited and the free activity of intelligence may be limited for the whole of the subject's lifetime …
> In a second type the intellectual development is sufficiently strong to resist the sexual repression which has hold of it … Here investigation becomes a sexual activity, often the exclusive one, and the feeling that comes from settling things in one's mind and explaining them replaces sexual satisfaction; third type, which is the rarest and most perfect, escapes both inhibition of thought and neurotic compulsive thinking … the libido evades the fate of repression by being sublimated from the very beginning into curiosity and by becoming attached to the powerful instinct for research as a reinforcement. (1910c, p. 79)

Three examples of sex education

Patient A. related that she had asked her father how babies are made. He answered that when a man and woman love each other very much, they go to bed and make love, out of which results a baby. This very vague explanation did not satisfy her, and she queried her grandmother, who gave her a protracted and thorough explanation of bees, flowers, and fertilisation—which also did not answer her questions. Only at the age of nine, when she was filling out a homework assignment on the differences between male and female bodies with her parents' help, did she understand the connections and explanations of fertilisation and birth. This time, her parents were forced to help her in this realisation. When her grandmother heard about this, she became quite upset and wanted to "correct" A.'s new explanations. Now, A. was confident enough to laughingly tell her grandmother she had already learned the correct version at school.

Interpretation

The patient's father responded to her questions, but in such a fashion that she neither became enlightened nor dared to ask further questions. Everything was vague, and she ended up feeling stupid and ignorant. In general, thinking was discouraged in their family. Her father—loving and friendly during the week—got drunk every Friday, demolishing the icebox and kitchen appliances, shouting until he fell asleep on the floor. The patient never dared to look into her family's situation or confront her father. Inhibited curiosity and diminished intelligence could be assessed in this patient: she remained on a primitive mental level, expressing her problems through massive psychosomatic symptoms that soon posed considerable problems for her, motivating her to enter analysis.

The question of sexual enlightenment cannot be taken out of the general family context and isolated.

Another patient, B., said she had noticed on holidays at her grandmother's farm that some eggs were fertilised and some not. She discussed with her friends what this could mean—whether every egg became a chicken and how seeds entered into the egg. At school, the children discussed this question avidly. My patient then decided she could ask the teacher, who was a nun. However, when B. posed the question in the middle of class, the nun reddened and said excitedly that she should sit down and never ask such impudent questions again. B., however, would not give up and continued her questioning. Her parents enlightened her through explanations of bees pollinating flowers. When her older sister first menstruated and asked her for advice, they were both convinced the sister was pregnant, since their brother had touched her one Sunday in the parents' bed. It was finally the maid who explained sexual matters to the two confused girls. B. was only truly informed by her fiancé, whom she married at eighteen—a virgin.

Interpretation

Although patient B. also received no adequate answers to her questions, she did not give up. She discussed sex with her friends and sisters, and considered this legitimate. She attempted to obtain information from other people. Her family was clearly structured; there was considerable rivalry between the siblings, but also a good sense of solidarity. She was able to sustain her curiosity and thirst for knowledge, becoming a good student and a self-motivated, prolific reader.

Often, important information on sex comes from siblings, friends, or babysitters; here, half-truths and distortions are often propagated, leading to lifelong confusion and irritations. A third example:

> In a workshop with Isca Salzberger-Wittenberg, one teacher told of a female student who bothered the class with her interminable questions. It seemed impossible to satisfy her with any answer. The seminar leader's comment to this was: "Then she must not be getting the right answers, she must want to know answers to life's big questions!" At the next seminar meeting, the teacher said she had called a parents' evening in order to inform them of her plan to speak about anatomical sex differences, birth, and pregnancy in a two-hour session. Since it was a private Catholic school, she emphasised that parents were free to keep their child home from school that day if they opposed having a teacher enlighten the class on this topic. The teacher also invited a doctor, who was herself in the last stage of pregnancy. The mother of the child who asked so many questions said her child was absolutely not interested in sexual matters, and would remain at home that day. The child, however, did attend the session, posing a number of intelligent questions that were answered openly and clearly. The children were also allowed to touch the pregnant doctor's belly and feel the baby's movements. To the teacher's great surprise, the child seemed satisfied afterwards and could concentrate again on her lessons, now only posing relevant questions. The child's mother was completely surprised at her daughter's sexual curiosity, mentioning incidentally that she herself was four months pregnant.

It often surprises non-psychoanalysts how often these concepts can be applied in daily life and how helpful they are. The diversion of sexual curiosity to other areas cannot be satisfied when urgent questions remain unanswered or when the answers are confusing. The insight that sex education is a significant component of education is now commonly accepted, and it is offered in school to inform children if it was not previously provided at home.

Developmental theory in Klein and Bion

Melanie Klein

One could say that Melanie Klein supplemented Freud's vertical structures of conscious, preconscious, and unconscious levels with a horizontal level—the relationship to an object, that is, to another person—which is why this direction in psychoanalysis is also called "object relations theory". Klein directed the psychoanalytic perspective towards the development of object relationships, in this case the early relationship between mother and baby. She assumed that the baby has a rudimentary core ego from birth on, which seeks a relationship to an object, to the mother. This biological basis of behaviour is inborn. In point of fact, we can observe (either live or on video recordings) how babies actively seek visual contact with their mothers after birth. Other forms of initial contact include skin contact and recognition of the mother's smell. We assume that along with this contact to the mother's skin, perception of her voice and gaze, the baby also perceives her inner feelings; similarly, we assume that a baby's emotional mood influences his perception of the world. Five days after birth, babies are already able to distinguish the smell of their mother's milk from other mothers' (Diem-Wille, 2013). If the mother or father can develop psychic space for their relationship to the baby, the baby will feel accepted in a stable relationship. A special form of unconscious communication occurs when the baby projects parts of himself—a part he experiences as unbearable—into another person, his mother, or "introjects" parts of his mother into himself. Klein thus extends the Freudian concept of identification, postulating—through the images of introjection and projection—the creation of an inner world from the time of birth on. The ego "has an orientation outwards and inwards … with a constant fluctuation between internal and external objects and situations" (Klein, 1945, p. 22). Klein calls this system of unconscious primitive communication "projective identification" (Klein, 1946). According to Heinz Weiss, "In this way, Klein described the relationship between inner world and outer reality as a *constant exchange*, where both unconscious fantasies and the mediators are formed as well as undergoing themselves continual modification" (2013, p. 910). Klein borrows the metaphor of a carrier pigeon carrying a message from one person's inner world to the other's, in order to describe traversing the distance between the child's and the mother's inner worlds. Klein thus extends Freud's concept of unconscious fantasies establishing not only the structure and negotiation of the inner world, but also the "matrix of inter-subjective relationships" (ibid., p. 903).

Klein also extends our understanding of the learning process, by emphasising the relationship between two emotionally linked persons. Instead of putting attention on the child isolated from her most intimate human relationship, focus is on the conscious and unconscious exchange between mother and baby. Whether a child can develop interest in the world, examining objects with curiosity, depends on adequate attention given her in her first human relationship: if that person could help the child through the first turbulent years of life, bearing her psychic pain and joy, desires and fantasised fears of punishment, then the child can build upon a stable, sturdy relationship. If early experiences have been only inadequately mastered, conflicts will erupt at the outset of latency—manifested in problems of learning and concentration, separation anxiety in attending school, or violent behaviour.

Wilfred Bion

In order to further understand these forms of relationship and unconscious communication, Wilfred Bion constructed—on the basis of Melanie Klein's projective identification—a model of "container and contained" which I will now briefly summarise. Bion distinguishes between pathological and normal forms of projective identification. The normal form is founded in Bion's understanding of the earliest and most primitive prelinguistic communication processes, which occur for the most part unconsciously. Along with Freud, we could say that the child's unconscious communicates directly with the mother's unconscious, without the conscious level being involved. Both Freud and Bion see this process of emotional exchange as analogous to a physical process of exchange: ingestion of food, love, and attention, physical and psychological digestion, and the excretion of digestive products—both on the physical and psychic levels.

In the 1950s, Bion developed a "theory of thinking" which seeks to explain the development of thought processes—a theory that has exerted a significant influence on subsequent psychoanalytical theory and clinical work. In this model, Bion attempts to comprehend both normal early communication and also the fragmented thinking of psychotic patients, whereby he proposes three models for understanding the process of thinking (Spillius, 1988, p. 154).

The *first model* centres on unconscious fantasy, in Bion's formulation a "preconception" used to test reality. Similarly to Kant, who postulated a priori views of space and time enabling thought, Bion (1962) assumes the foreknowledge of an emotional bond between subject and object, whose *Urform* (or prototype) is embodied in the fit between an infant's mouth and mother's nipple. The child seeks to discover whether his inborn disposition can find the kind of match that his mouth found in the nipple. Does the fantasy of an inborn opinion (preconception) find a parallel in the realisation of this fantasy? According to Bion, in order to proceed from the conception of the breast to a thought, an experience or "actualisation"—that is, the experience of a real breast—is required, and this experience together with the preconception breast-mouth results in a kind of thought. Bion assumes that there exists an inborn expectation of a link between two objects, between nipple and mouth and between penis and vagina. Under adequate inner and outer conditions, the baby can tolerate short-term absence, and the baby's preconception can forge a link to a "negative realisation" (an absent breast or a frustration), in order to become a "thought of the breast". Bion writes:

> Is a "thought" the same as an absence of a thing? If there is no "thing", is "no thing" a thought and is it by virtue of the fact that there is "no thing" that one recognizes that "it" must be a thought? (1962, p. 35)

Klein emphasised that in the paranoid-schizoid position, an absent (part) object is experienced as a bad object. In Bion's scheme, however, the experience of the absent breast can constitute the precondition for a thought that helps the child to wait until the good breast arrives again. Spillius points out "[T]his development of an ability to think bridges the gap between need and satisfaction and thus makes frustration more tolerable ..." (2011, p. 509). At this juncture, a positive circle is put into motion within the child's psyche. Slowly, the capacity to think arises: the child thinks that a bad feeling arises because the good object is absent, but it can return. When a child can tolerate frustrations as well as positive or negative experiences, this creates a basis for learning from experience. But if the child cannot tolerate frustration or has only a limited capacity for doing so, he will also be unable to bear a bad feeling and must expel it.

The second model is centred on how the baby deals with frustration or negative reality, when there is no breast to satisfy hunger. How the child deals with this depends on her capacity for dealing with frustration. Klein believed that the "absent breast" was experienced by the child as a bad breast, since the unconscious knows no negation. Bion extended this thought. The absence of a loved object induces an emotional experience Bion considered the starting point for thinking—since a hallucinatory wish-fulfilment occurs in fantasy (Freud, 1900a, p. 539) in order for the thinker to satisfy his wishes. Ferenczi (1924) assumed that a newborn baby, sated in his first sleep, believes himself once more in his former form of existence—in other words, dreams himself back to his mother's womb. If the child is able to bear frustration, the frustration over an absent breast can transform itself into a thought. In thinking, the child can make contact with his fears, gradually recognising that he is frustrated because the good object is currently absent and may or may not return.

However, if the child is not able to tolerate the frustration of an absent object, the thought of transforming the bad object into an absent good object is no longer possible; instead, the child experiences a concrete bad object and expels it through omnipotent projection. This vitiates the development of thought and symbolisation.

The third model comprises Bion's theory of the "container and contained". Taking up Klein's concept of projective identification, Bion nevertheless makes a distinction between normal and pathological projective identification.

In his psychoanalytic work with psychotic patients, Bion discovered that they made statements they themselves did not understand. He considered his task as psychoanalyst to make something of this "incoherent stuff". Based on Melanie Klein's ideas, Bion developed the concept of infantile mental development. Bion believed that the baby has feelings or needs, emerging from the inside or outside, with which she cannot cope. It attempts to expel—to breathe out, to scream out, to urinate out—the part of herself affected by these sensations from her body. Bion (1962) terms such sensations "beta elements". Where do these projected experiences go? It is clear that without modification of these raw feelings, no development or emotional growth can take place. The child behaves in such a way that she evokes those feelings she desires to be rid of in the mother. The projective identification is an omnipotent fantasy, but it leads to a behaviour that calls forth the same sensations in the mother. If the mother is emotionally stable and empathetic, she can take up these sensations (beta elements) emotionally and be touched by them, assuming and modifying them through her understanding in accordance with her emotional capacity. In this context, Winnicott (1956) speaks of a "primary maternal preoccupation", called "reverie" by Bion—a kind of dreamy intuition. This attitude is not a faculty of the mother alone, but rather a common activity between mother and baby to the advantage of both. How the mother deals with these projected feelings is comparable to a mental "digestion" of the baby's raw feelings. The mother thus becomes a container for the baby's fragmented experience. This mental activity of the mother is unconscious, and is compared by Riesenberg-Malcolm (2001) to those birds which first masticate their babies' food and then place it in their beaks. The baby does not only ingest these experiences (as put into words), but also the manner in which her mother perceives the task of intellectual digestion. Bion calls this "digested" form of experience that the baby can then introject "alpha elements". They are the foundations for learning from experience, of reality-bound knowledge. Bion calls the capability to transform beta elements into alpha elements the "alpha function" of the mother. The child can then not only introject the transformed alpha elements, but also (slowly) introject the very function of transformation. In this way, she acquires the incipient capacity to bear frustration and to think.

If the mother, however, is so concentrated on her own turbulent feelings that she cannot take in the baby's expelled experiences, thus denying the baby access and not understanding it, these feelings rebound back to the baby, overwhelming him. Or containment does not take place, due to the child's intolerance and envy that the mother is able to do something he cannot. The child cannot take those experiences in, and feels empty and flat (lack of containment). Moreover, if the mother is overwhelmed by her feelings of dejection, aggression, abandonment, or unhappiness, she not only refuses the projected feelings, but also presses her feelings into the baby (parasitic containment). The overwhelmed baby then expresses this through somatic problems.

The same function assumed by the mother when she mentally "digests" the baby's raw feelings is also assumed by the analyst in therapy—attempting to take in the patient's words in their raw form and interpret them in a manner coherent and comprehensible to the patient. De Masi (2003) points out that Bion's view of the unconscious as a function that transforms thoughts and feelings (the emotional unconscious) preceded neuroscientific theories. He writes: "Thus, startlingly, Bion anticipated the neuroscientific theory of the unconscious, which ascribes to it the function of working through feelings" (p. 15).

This concept of "containment"—the transformation of undigested beta elements into alpha elements—is included by many schools of psychology as a valuable element of theory. For the topic of maternal thinking, the container-contained model has brought theories of thinking and feeling closer together. In his introduction to his chapter "Theory of Thinking in 'Melanie Klein Today'", Spillius points out how this link can be made: "containment" describes how feelings acquire meaning and how the capability to think develops:

> In "A Theory of Thinking", and indeed in his later work, Bion did not do as much as he might have to link his three models. It is surely repeated experiences of alternations between positive and negative realizations that encourage the development of thoughts and thinking. And the return of an absent mother gives rise to a particularly important instance, repeated many times in childhood (and in an analysis), of a mother taking in and transforming, or failing to transform, the bad-breast-present experience. (1988, p. 156)

How can these theories be confirmed or refuted through observing a child with his parents? It must once again be emphasised that the basic pattern of the child's personality is formed out of the experience of being nurtured by an understanding person (mother or father) in the early years. Later experiences rest on this foundation. Here are three examples of this taken from different experiences.

Case studies from latency

Winston Churchill, who in his autobiography writes of his early child-hood, describes with particular eloquence his first day at school, sup-plying a good illustration of the effects of misunderstanding a child's emotional and cognitive situation. Winston Churchill grew up in Ireland, where his education was mostly in the hands of his trusted governess Mrs. Everest. (Her picture was hung on the wall of his study in the Cab-inet War Rooms, the underground command centre in London during the Blitz). Indeed, Mrs. Everest was more a confidante for little Winston than his mother was, although he admired his mother rather like the evening star—from a distance. At the age of seven, he was meant to start school; he characterises himself as a "troublesome child"—fearful, easily upset, but full of hope at getting the chance to play with children his age. The school his parents had selected was an exclusive private school; there were only ten pupils per class, expensive accoutrements, and beautiful sports facilities. The term had already begun when his mother brought him to school. They drank tea with the headmaster, with Winston afraid to make a bad impression.

> When the last sound of my mother's departing wheels had died away, the Headmaster invited me to hand over any money I had in my possession. I produced my three half-crowns, which were duly entered in a book … Then we quitted the Headmaster's parlour and the comfortable private side of the house, and entered the more bleak apartments reserved for the instruction and accommodation of the pupils. I was taken into a Form Room and told to sit at a desk. All the other boys were out of doors, and I was alone with the Form Master. He produced a thin greeny-brown, covered book filled with words in different types of print.
>
> "You have never done any Latin before, have you?" he said.
>
> "No, sir."
>
> "This is a Latin grammar." He opened it at a well-thumbed page. "You must learn this," he said, pointing to a number of words in a frame of lines. "I will come back in half an hour and see what you know."
>
> Behold me then on a gloomy evening, with an aching heart, seated in front of the First Declension.
>
> Mensa a table

Mensa O table

Mensam a table

Mensae of a table

Mensae to or for a table

Mensa by, with or from a table

What on earth did it mean? Where was the sense in it? It seemed absolute rigmarole to me. However, there was one thing I could always do: I could learn by heart. And I thereupon proceeded, as far as my private sorrows would allow, to memorise the acrostic-looking task which had been set me.

In due course the Master returned.

"Have you learnt it?" he asked.

"I think I can *say* it, sir," I replied; and I gabbled it off.

He seemed so satisfied with this that I was emboldened to ask a question.

"What does it mean, sir?"

"It means what it says. Mensa, a table. Mensa is a noun of the First Declension. There are five declensions. You have learnt the singular of the First Declension."

"But," I repeated, "What does it mean?"

"Mensa means a table," he answered.

"Then why does mensa also mean O table," I enquired, "and what does O table mean?"

"Mensa, O table, is the vocative case," he replied.

"But why O table?" I persisted in genuine curiosity.

"O table,—you would use that in addressing a table, in invoking a table." And then seeing he was not carrying me with him, "You would use it in speaking to a table."

"But I never do," I blurted out in honest amazement.

"If you are impertinent, you will be punished, and punished, let me tell you, very severely," was his conclusive rejoinder. (1930, p. 25)

This experience set the paradigm for Winston's attitude to studying; he in fact did not study, and was punished cruelly for this. He was publicly beaten again and again, and began to lisp and stutter. He continues in his autobiography:

The Form Master's observations about punishment were by no means without their warrant at St. James' School. Flogging with the birch in accordance with the Eton fashion was a great feature in its curriculum. But I am sure no Eton boy, and certainly no Harrow boy of my day, ever received such a cruel flogging as this Headmaster was accustomed to inflict upon the little boys who were in his care and power. They exceeded in severity anything that would be tolerated in any of the Reformatories under the Home Office. My reading in later life has supplied me with some possible explanations of his temperament. (ibid., p. 26)

Interpretation

The setting for Winston's school experiences was unfavourable. He did not begin school simultaneously with the other children; he missed the starting ritual, the gradual acquaintance with other pupils; in the first year, when all pupils come together for the first time, they can get to know one another. We know that the first contacts between pupils-- but also between adults, for example in seminars—are characterised by chance conversations and meetings, but often lead to long friendships. Presumably, the brusque behaviour of the headmaster and Latin teacher also expressed their annoyance that this prominent child did not keep to the common rules and demands. Their treatment of him was tantamount to punishment; instead of letting him play with the other children, introducing them and letting them greet one another, they separated him from the others and assigned him a kind of punitive exercise. Without any introduction and guidance to learning an ancient language, he was confronted with the rote learning of grammar. His good memory and quick understanding allowed him to complete the exercises swiftly, but at the same time he conceived a deeply entrenched aversion to ancient languages.

Nobody responded to his feelings, to his fear, his feeling of being lost, and presumably his homesickness. Instead of showing him the house, his room, and his fellow pupils, the schoolmaster brought him alone to a room, where he listened longingly to the sounds of other children playing. Winston was not intimidated; he tried to understand his situation and posed questions. Presumably he was expressing his wish to orient himself in a new environment. The communication between him and the Latin teacher is itself like the ostensible conversation with a wooden table that is incapable of supplying an adequate answer. The two speak past one another—even worse, each feels provoked by the other. The Latin teacher was annoyed because he considered the boy's questions impudent. Only when he threatened to punish Winston did Winston stop asking questions. The boy must have felt helpless and misunderstood, lonely and lost. There was not even a minimal form of communication, no approach made towards his emotional situation. Apparently Winston managed to annoy the head, because an immediate enmity arose from this meeting. Later, Winston also stepped on the man's straw hat and was severely punished once again; the boy seemed to be a master of provocation. We might prefer to see Winston as a victim of the cruel school system, but we know that such intense victim-oppressor relationships are nourished from both sides. The victim secretly feels himself powerful, setting his torturer into such a rage that he loses his control. In the meantime, Winston extended his denial to ancient languages, mathematics, and biology.

How urgently Winston would have needed a sympathetic teacher who could take in his turbulent feelings of fear, hope, and manifold separation anxiety vis-à-vis parents, governess, and Ireland itself. Nobody took up the chance to forge a special relationship with the new child. Tragically, Winston extended his feeling of exclusion to the entire school, to learning, and the other pupils. He hated the school and yet had to spend two years there. Only a severe case of double pneumonia caused his parents to withdraw him from school. He only confided his desperation to his governess, and the parents failed to see behind the façade of the brave little boy. In intrapsychic terms, we can understand his truculent attitude as a struggle, where not giving in is an answer to terror.

> Where my reason, imagination or interest were not engaged, I would not or I could not learn. My teachers saw me at once backward and precocious, reading books beyond my years and yet at the bottom of the Form. They were offended. (ibid., p. 27)

His description of the distance between him and his fellow pupils indicates that his arrogant attitude was merely a defence against helplessness and desperation. In his article "On Arrogance" (1957), Bion describes this defensive attitude that attempts to preserve a fragile balance through denigrating others, onto whom the individual projects her own helplessness. Nobody (not even the person herself) must recognise how delicate and fragile, desperate and lonely she feels. The others in her environment seem small and unimportant, stupid and worthless—an effect of projective identification. In contrast to Bion's patient, Winston presumably exhibits a mild case of arrogance as defence. In the scene described above, we see the child seeking understanding and still posing questions; nobody understands his emotional situation.

Winston was transferred to a small school in Brighton, run by two ladies, where there was an element of "kindness and of sympathy".

Truculence also constitutes a protection towards surviving unbearable situations. In Churchill's case, this defensive form of arrogance only occurred in mild form, tempered by his stubbornness and his extraordinary intellectual and rhetorical talents, as well as his sharp humour. The preservation of an intellectual attitude in latency—with negative aspects of denial, stubbornness, and a monomaniacal desire to conquer fields of knowledge—also constitutes a great strength. Winston's courage and his ability to get through these terrible school years were later transformed into resistance against Nazi Germany, as a fighting slogan for the entire British Empire. In his famous 1940 speech just after being named prime minister, Churchill thus only promised "blood, toil, tears and sweat"; in the early war years, where Great Britain resolutely fought Hitler without any allies: "We will never surrender. We will fight them on the beaches; we will fight them in the streets. We will never surrender!"

Churchill's biographer Sebastian Haffner (2012) writes how Churchill managed to survive alone at the age of seven—far too early—with an inimical school against him. In the bitter war years of 1940–41, he managed to preserve and stoke the British fighting spirit without allies, and then win over the USA as an ally.

An example from pedagogical practice

The case of twelve-year-old James Frost (not his real name) and his teacher Ms H. is an example from pedagogical practice. The teacher succeeded in integrating this very disturbed and aggressive child, who was no longer willing to attend school, into the class. I would like to direct special attention to Ms H.'s psychoanalytic attitude underlying her pedagogical practice, as distinct from therapy. In her dealings with James's parents and grandparents, however, Ms H. could then clearly demonstrate the necessity for therapeutic help for the child, so that James finally did receive psychotherapy parallel to her work with him.

Family and school background

James is twelve years old. Due to his emotional and social problems, he was deemed in need of special education; for this reason, a second teacher—Ms H.—was assigned to him. His parents were divorced when he was three years old. The grandmother relates that James's mother clung to him after her divorce, and was unable to set limits. This initial information on James's first years of life indicates that the roots of his psychic problems must lie in those first years. When his mother began a new relationship with another man, James was seven, and behaved very rebelliously towards him. When he found out his mother was pregnant, he came at her with a knife; her boyfriend took the knife away from James. After this, James's maternal grandmother agreed to take the boy in.

At elementary school, James had already once been placed in a psychiatric clinic for five months, which was a terrible experience for him. He now threatens to kill himself if put back there. At the time, he was in psychotherapy, but soon broke it off and since then refuses to go to a psychiatrist or psychotherapist. Only Ms H. has been able to motivate James to accept a psychotherapist's help.

James's mother had a second baby; at the beginning of Ms H.'s work with James, this half-brother is two and a half years old. Since being released from the psychiatric clinic, James lives with his maternal grandmother.

In 2009, James entered year five. However, after five months he was again sent to a psychiatric clinic for trying to strangle another student and physically attacking the teacher who was attempting to separate them.

Ms H., who discussed her work with James in the Work Discussion Group (Rustin, 2008)—the form of Work Discussion Group developed by Martha Harris seeks to contribute to work situations through psychoanalytic thinking—works as a teacher in year five. There are six children with special education needs in her class.

Spring 2010

James stays home from school before the ski course; his grandmother is beside herself, since he supplies no reason for refusing to go to school. When the ski course begins, however, he participates in it and behaves normally the entire time. After the ski course is over, he once again stays home. His grandmother contacts Ms H., who is requested by the school principal to comply with the grandmother's wish that James receive a home visit. In this conversation Ms H. learns that James retreats with a friend to a secret place in the wetlands, to which he has also led his grandmother and shown her his treasure—a large bone. Ms H. manages to engage James in conversation through discussing this bone, which is apparently from a bear. During the conversation, the teacher observes not only James's feelings, but also her own, in order to see whether he might be unconsciously projecting his feelings into her in order that she understand him better. The conversation centres on James's interest in archeological digs; he talks about a book on archaeology, and also a television film.

The next day, James once again is absent from school, and some days later his grandmother informs the teachers that "something terrible has happened". James has "attacked" her again, and the police have arrived. Ms H. is very upset, but establishes to herself that she is not responsible for this development and decides to wait before she reacts.

The day after that, James's mother calls up the school and informs them that he will now live with her (with her husband and James's two-and-a-half-year-old half-brother). During the next two weeks (until the end of April), James attends school; then, without prior notice, he stops coming. A new crisis arises: James refuses to get out of bed, as his mother reports. He also is missing from school the whole of May. The social worker suggests foster care, but James reacts extremely negatively to this, threatening suicide in a quite convincing manner. In a discussion on May 20, 2010, the mother pleads with the teacher to "bring James through this school year without him having to repeat it".

Discussion I

In her account, the teacher indicates what enormous emotional pressure is on her, as well as the pressure on James's mother. On the one hand, Ms H. has doubts as to whether she can help such a disturbed child; on the other hand, she has managed to build a stable emotional relationship with James, which makes her more confident of helping him.

It is important at the outset to give the teacher space to express her feelings and fears. It seems an optimistic sign that James can establish emotional contact to the teacher: he agreed to speak with her at his grandmother's house. The ensuing conversation enables the teacher to discover James's interest in archaeology.

We can see both the psychoanalytic perspective and the capacity for containment: here, Ms H. and the group see not only James's disturbed aspects, but wish to come into contact with his healthy side. Early emotional disturbances that only become visible in latency or puberty seem especially alarming to observers, since infantile, primitive feelings are being expressed not by a two year old but instead by a ten or twelve year old. For the teacher, it constitutes a relief to see James's reaction as an expression of early emotional conflicts. James expressed that he would like to speak with Ms H, which we understand as showing a trusting, stable relationship. In the further course of events, we see that Ms H.'s readiness to work with James is a major factor in his being allowed to remain in school.

A further point of discussion revolves around encouraging the mother to organise professional therapeutic help for James, and emphasising that the social worker must remain responsible for managing his social care. On reflection, it is emphasised how important it is for Ms H. to clearly set limits of responsibility, both vis-à-vis the other responsible parties and—as is even more important—herself. The limiting of the task allotted to her also lessens her fear of being overwhelmed by this difficult "case". The teacher's job consists of supporting the mother and grandmother in the attempt to bring James once more into contact with the school. He is meant to see that he must achieve something if he is to finish the school year.

At this point, we shall observe concretely how Ms H. deals with James through two discussions from the Work Discussion Group.

> In the meantime, two weeks have gone by. James's mother and I talk on the phone every morning at 7:45, with the same result: James will not get up. I report this to the principal, who relays it to the district school council and the youth social agency.
>
> By now, James has been missing all of May. Ms Frost requests a meeting with me and we meet in front of the conference room. She has a firm handshake, but I think I see discouragement in her eyes ... She breathes in audibly and says that she is at the end of her resources. James is sweet and good at home, but wants nothing to do with school. He can't stand two of his teachers—they only sit up front and do nothing ... James likes a third teacher, Mr. Z., who hands the pupils' assignments back on the next day. I do not

comment on these remarks, but I mention that Mr. Z. and Mr. B., who instruct James in two subjects, are quite firm teachers, not as friendly and calm as Mr. L. "James's father was also calm and patient," answers Ms Frost. "Maybe Mr. L. is like James's father? And James doesn't like being reminded."

"Maybe so, maybe he doesn't like some of his teachers, Ms Frost. But how will he do his schoolwork and end the school year positively? How do you want to motivate him to come to school?" I ask.

At this point, Ms Frost avoids my questioning and tells about the lady from the social agency who advised her to put James into foster care. She absolutely does not want this, she says with strong emphasis ... I want to know if she has already spoken with James about this option. "Yes," she answers, with her shoulders sinking forward, "then he would kill himself." She makes an unhappy and enervated impression on me. She cowers opposite me with her hands gripping each other, her eyes seemingly fixed on me in a search for help. Her sole goal would be to get James through this school year without him having to repeat it ... She is counting on the tutoring he could have during vacation. My eyes must have expressed scepticism, for Ms Frost evidently has limited herself to this one goal.

In the Work Discussion Group, Ms H. said she has discovered that there is no proportion of school days required for a pupil to participate in instruction. She says she will investigate which of James's teachers is qualified to make an evaluation of him and which examinations James would have to take.

"'What does James do all day?' I enquire. His mother reports that he is bored—he has to accompany her everywhere and is not allowed to sit alone and play computer games. Indeed, there is no doubt that he is bored."

Ms H. eventually finds out that he has three examinations left: in biology, history, and geography.

Discussion II

This precise recounting of the conversation demonstrates how important it would be for James (and his mother) to remain in school and complete the school year. (Later, Ms H. also visited James at home, where

James showed her the bone he had unearthed. They then discussed archaeological digs, which James had researched on the internet.) For James's mother, this conversation must have represented a great relief—the experience of hearing not reproach, but understanding and support. She then was able to take James back into her family and wants to keep him there instead of sending him elsewhere, which indicates a positive prognosis.

In discussion, someone has the idea of motivating James to complete his written assignments by email. Ms H. believes that since he is a very intelligent boy, his inactivity must be boring for him and that he would be perfectly capable of achieving well—especially if his achievements were then afforded recognition.

In the class conference, it is officially decided to take up Ms H.'s suggestion and let James graduate from this year—he has written at least one paper in every subject and also has shown enough other accomplishments. This constitutes a win-win situation for everyone involved.

Email contact

The following emails were exchanged:

From Ms H. to Ms Frost:

Good evening, Ms Frost!

I hope James is already under less pressure, since he has now been considered eligible for evaluation. Still, I consider it necessary for him to show a certain achievement if he is to receive a diploma this year. Without more of his active work, his diploma would be devalued, as would the achievements he has already made. So I think it would be a good idea to use the Internet as a medium. James could work on a chapter he selects, for instance in biology, at the computer and then send it in ... I find it important that he makes contact to the school.

James's mother answered back the same day, saying that James was willing to work at the computer. Five days later, on Sunday, James sent in (through his mother) three excellent assignments. His mother wrote:

I let him work completely independently and hardly interfered at all. He did of course use phrases from other texts, but not simply "copied in". Please send it on to the appropriate teachers ...

James selected the following themes: "sharks" for biology, "volcanoes" for geography, and "Pompeii" for history.

On Monday, Ms H. writes back: the teachers have—independently from one another—given James's papers As; in the class conference, it was decided to let James graduate on from the class. Other requirements in maths, German, and English were specified, and James is also allowed to send these assignments in on a DVD, which he proceeded to do.

Discussion III

In the group, Ms H. tells of her surprise at Ms Frost's immediate and compliant reaction. The group discusses whether James and his mother might be relieved that now an actual accomplishment is expected of him. It seems as if they both were waiting for this.

The themes James has chosen in the three requisite subjects afford a view into his stormy inner world. In biology, he chooses "sharks" and in geography "volcanoes", both of which point to eruptive danger and/ or oral aggression (biting). His interest in Pompeii can be understood as an unconscious indication of his wish for someone to take an interest in the contents of his ruined inner world. From this vantage point, James's work, in its childlike sobriety, constitutes a meaningful treatment of these themes.

Seeing these themes as an expression of James's threatening inner state helps to understand why he feels unable to come to school at this time. Presumably, he is afraid to explode, to bite, or to reveal his hidden secrets. Fear of these primitive feelings accordingly points to the infantile roots of the early malady revealed in his "baby component".

For James's teachers and fellow students, it is important to experience that he can complete a scholastic accomplishment even though he has psychic problems. The teacher informed the class that James cannot attend school at the moment because he has a psychic illness "that we don't see", adding that she hopes he can come back next year.

For Ms H., it constitutes a relief that James hands in his assignments and that he is required to study the same things as the other pupils. For everyone involved, it is important that they can go about "business as usual"; this affords them structure and security, and diminishes the distance not only between James and the teachers but between him and the other children—the distance caused by his absence from school.

The integrative success James attained by handing his assignments in via email is demonstrated by the fact that—to the teacher's surprise—he felt able to pick up his diploma in person on the last day of school.

By chance, Ms H. had met James and his mother, and suggested he pick up his diploma at school. She was certain he would not take her up on this suggestion, and was amazed to see him suddenly in the classroom. There was no seat for him—but another pupil brought over a chair.

In the group, it was pointed out that the teacher had underestimated the significance of her "containing" intervention. Through his appearance at school, James demonstrated that he felt part of the class.

School year 2010/11

In the next school year, James attended school unwillingly at his mother's urging, but could be motivated towards more participation. He is a good to excellent student and completes all his written assignments. There are many reports on his leaving class and discussions where he

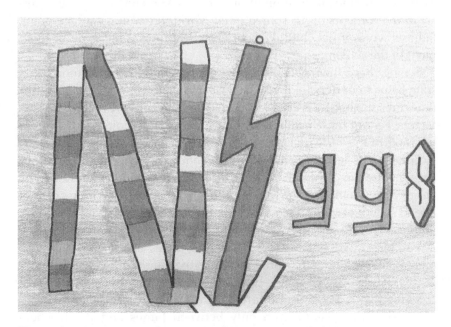

Illustration 10. James's drawing "NOTHING" ("NICHTS").

begins to cry, since he feels so miserable and hopeless. Ms H. made an important contribution by communicating to the other teachers that James's passivity, refusal, and absence was not directed against them personally but was rather an expression of his desperation and inner turbulence. Now, I will describe a typical intervention of Ms H. that made it possible for James to understand and overcome his total refusal and resistance.

Report

> In drawing class, James sits before the empty table. After a few minutes, I try to motivate him to draw something. He only shakes his head. After five more minutes, I start again: "Would you like to draw me NOTHING?" James gives me a look that I interpret as incomprehension. "You could draw or write NOTHING on the piece of paper; maybe with special colours, weird letters." "Wow," says another child sitting next to us, "can I do that too?" "Sure, you're almost done with your assignment anyway. If you go back to it afterwards, you can also do NOTHING now." Both boys grin and begin immediately to discuss their ideas. I go away and give other children tips or praise their good ideas. From the corner of my eye, I can see the two boys drawing something while they talk enthusiastically.

Discussion IV

Ms H. has had a simple but inspired idea. She understands James's refusal to draw as "resistance", goes along with this, and makes it the subject of the drawing exercise. James is surprised when she tells him to draw "nothing". The fact that he then complies shows that James has a very good relationship with Ms H. In his drawing, James uses colours; he creates a clear structure and decorates it with patterns. With such a disturbed child, the use of colours indicates a lessening of depression; he is able to achieve a creative accomplishment, which motivates his neighbour to make a similar drawing. In this intervention, Ms H. shows him a way to participate in the lesson and express his mood in the drawing: his desire to do "nothing" and his conviction that he is incapable of doing anything. With his neighbour's participation, a collaboration ensues—supplanting his former isolation.

Indeed, James now begins to make contact to two other boys and to speak with them. His clothing, which was exclusively black this last year, begins to become somewhat more colourful.

This seemingly simple intervention is an excellent example of how the psychoanalytic approach enables us to understand a child at a deeper level. The teacher has succeeded in her primary task—motivating James to shape his feelings creatively. Almost incidentally, she creates a space where James can express his rebellion and simultaneously feels understood.

The fixed setting here—that is, the drawing lesson—gives both James and the teacher security and stability.

In conclusion, here is a short excerpt from the Work Discussion Group's report:

> One hour later, James is working in shop class without complaint. He accepts tips; he asks what he should do with the project they are working on. He can bear my physical proximity. He looks in my eyes when I approach him, and signalises interest (I believe). He does not become fearful when my fingers touch his while we hold the piece together. He listens attentively when I give him directions for using the tool, and then attempts to implement them. James seeks out my eyes and obviously is waiting for my confirming nod. There are no conflicts between the boys, they are easy to motivate and take pleasure in the work process ... the two hours pass swiftly, James works without being requested to.

In the reports, Ms H. describes precisely how she observes James, how he reacts to her comments, whether he can maintain eye contact with her. (James's further development will be described in my forthcoming book on adolescence.)

Forms of thought organisation according to Piaget

Jean Piaget's genetic theories of intelligence and thinking supply a complement to the psychoanalytic approach. Fatke (2010) contends that as a self-styled "system constructor", Piaget revolutionised our understanding of intellectual development from the first years of life through adolescence. Fatke positions Piaget next to Freud, who shed light on the dark areas of psychic events, the dynamics of the unconscious, and the formation of the psyche. Piaget (1983) developed a theory of stages in intellectual growth, comprising three interdependent stages in an unvarying order:

1. The sensorimotoric stage (0–2 years)
2. The stage of concrete operations, with two sub-stages:
   Preoperational stage (2–7 years)
   Concrete operational stage (7–11 years)
3. Formal operational stage, with two sub-stages:
   Organisational sub-stage (11–13 years)
   Sub-stage of achievement (15 years)

In the sensorimotoric stage, the child is centred on his own body, and slowly develops a blueprint for practical intelligence adapted to his environmental circumstances.

During the period of latency, the second sub-stage of stage two, concrete operational thought (7–11 years) and the first sub-stage of stage three, operational ordering (11–13 years) are relevant.

The stage of concrete operational thinking, according to Piaget, is "characterized by the beginnings of operational groupings in their various *concrete* forms and with their various forms of preservation" (1983, p. 66). Subsequently begins the "stage of the propositional-logical or formal operation … which subsumes other operations" (deduction, correlation, etc.) (ibid.).

Piaget considers the age of seven—which coincides in many countries with the beginning of school and thus the beginning of a new period of life—to be a "decisive turning point in intellectual development".

"With each complex aspect of psychic life, whether regarding intelligence or feelings, social relationships or purely individual activities, we can observe new forms of organization arise that conclude those accomplishments of the previous period and lend them a more stable balance, as well as constituting the foundation of an uninterrupted series of new constructions" (1964, p. 224).

As a proponent of genetic psychology, Piaget set himself the task of studying child intelligence and the development of perception according to the child's age. From describing the child's development and formation of her intellectual apparatus, he attempts to explain the nature and functioning of adult intelligence as well (ibid., p. 297). To obtain data for this, Piaget employed three methods: observation of children, experiment, and surveys or interviews.

Piaget describes the decisive developmental turning point from the small child (2–7 years) to the older child (7–12) as the stage of concrete operational intelligence, in accordance with three features:

- Intuition is now supplanted by the beginnings of logical thinking and rational operations
- Egocentric thinking is supplanted by general rules and measures
- Impulsive behaviour is supplanted by the beginnings of reflection.

From intuition to the beginning of logical thinking and rational operations

With the acquisition of language, the small child has—in addition to his merely sensorimotoric and practical intelligence, as Piaget termed it— also acquired the capability of describing his actions and reconstructing the past. Language deals with generalised concepts and insights, thus supporting individual thought with a comprehensive system of universal thought. However, the child cannot immediately adapt to this new reality; only slowly is his egocentrism supplanted by a thinking that is oriented to fellow human beings and reality. In latency, this capacity for logical thought enters a new phase.

Piaget conducted one famous experiment on children centring on liquid measurement. One container A and a narrower container B were shown to a child between four and six and a child between seven and eleven. A liquid is poured from a broader into a narrower but higher container. A five year old will say that the amount of water is different, with more water in the narrower container. A child of six and a half to seven years will say that the amount of water remains the same—and will point out that the second container is narrower and thus the water level higher. If a four- to six-year-old child is given an empty glass A and another empty, narrower glass B, and then asked to fill both glasses so that the same amount of water can be drunk from both, he will fill both glasses to the same height without considering their diameter. "The deeper reason for this oversight is that the small child only thinks about the *conditions*, neglecting the *transformations* as such" (ibid., pp. 262ff.). A latency child pours the same amount of water into both, even though the water level is higher in the narrower glass.

A similar experiment can be carried out using balls of modelling clay. A child of four to six is shown two balls of modelling clay of the same size (and duly asked to confirm this). Then, one ball is reshaped to a long sausage, and one into a short sausage. To the question of which sausage contains more clay, the child now points to the long sausage: "Of course, this one, it's longer." A seven-year-old child, however, answers the question correctly, seeing that both still have the same amount of clay. This means she has the capability of executing a "reversible operation". This capacity enables the latency child to develop a rational concept of space (order, constancy, distance, length, measure, etc.) and time (order, intervals), and carry out rational operations. The shift from intuition to operation is achieved when "two actions of the same type can be consolidated into a third, in turn belonging to this type, and immediately, these various functions can be reversed: thus, the act of unification (logical or arithmetic addition) is an operation, because various successive unifications become equivalent to one single unification (consolidated addition) and because unification can be reversed into separations (subtractions)" (ibid., p. 235).

Almost every child believes that a ball of clay, when reshaped into a sausage, remains "the same" clay—which Piaget calls "object permanence". The thought process entailed in recognising the constancy of a given quantity is very complex. It demands that the child recognise the transformation of the ball into a sausage of constant quantity, not being misled by the length of the sausage. Piaget describes this learning process in four stages:

1. First, the child only considers one dimension—for example, the length of the sausage. In eight out of ten cases, the child says the sausage contains more clay, since it is longer. In two out of ten cases, the child says the sausage is thinner, forgetting that it also has become longer.
2. When the child sees the sausage getting longer and longer as it is rolled out, the probability increases that she also observes the other dimension (thinness), then vacillating between one conclusion and the next.
3. When this happens, the probability increases that the child notices a correlation between both variations: in that when the sausage

becomes longer, it also becomes thinner. Piaget believes that now, the child's thinking has acquired a new quality: "He no longer is fixed on *configurations*, but instead begins to deal with *transformations*. The sausage is not simply 'long', it can 'lengthen' itself, etc." (1983, p. 111).

4. As soon as the child's thinking can consider transformations, the probability increases that he understands how a transformation can be reversed, also comparing these two transformations.

Thus, the child can make a further step in his cognitive development, since he has built concrete operational structures that are then further developed in puberty.

From egocentric thinking to consideration of general rules

The small child connects all her observations to herself; the child herself and her movements are seen as causing the movements of the heavens and stars. Piaget quotes several examples from his conversations with children:

PIAGET: Can the moon move where it wants to, or is there something moving it?

NAIN (FOUR AND
A HALF YEARS):   Yes, when I walk.

PIAGET: And when you walk?

NAIN: It comes with me, it follows me.

PIAGET: Does the moon move or not?

GAIMB (SEVEN):   It follows us.

PIAGET: Why?

GAIMB: When someone walks, it comes out.

PIAGET: Who makes the moon move?

GAIMB: We do.

PIAGET: How do we do that?

GAIMB: When someone walks. It moves all by itself …

PIAGET: If someone didn't move, would the moon move or not move?

GAIMB: The moon would stop moving.

PIAGET: And the sun?

GAIMB: It goes with us too.

The children are not bothered by the fact that people walk in different directions; they stick to their belief that they participate in the moon's movement and the magical attitude that "[W]e can command the heavens and the clouds, since their intentions are participating in ours" (Piaget, 1926, p. 138). Only later, when the child can detach himself from the centre of the world and understand the structuring of reality through reason—called by Piaget "rational assimilation"—does the child attribute to the heavens an independent existence.

Piaget describes the second and third stages regarding reality. In the second, the child cannot escape the contradiction that the moon moves but still cannot follow two people walking in opposite directions:

PIAGET ASKS SART
(FIVE YEARS,
   ELEVEN MONTHS): Does the moon move?
           SART: Yes.
         PIAGET: What happens, when you go for a walk?
           SART: You see it the whole time walking before you.
         PIAGET: Does it follow us or not?
           SART: It follows us, because it's fat.
         PIAGET: Does it go before us or not?
           SART: Yes.
         PIAGET: When the moon follows us, is it moving or not?
           SART: I don't know.

Sart cannot manage to make a synthesis; he thinks the moon is following us, while simultaneously believing it is not moving.

Piaget also describes the third phase, where the child sees through the illusion:

PIAGET ASKS PEC
   (SEVEN YEARS,
   THREE MONTHS): Is the moon moving when you go for a walk at night?
            PEC: It is far away, so you would say it's moving forward, but it isn't.
            KUF: When you walk, you would say that the moon is following, because it is big.
         PIAGET: And does it follow us?

> KUF: No—earlier I thought it was following us and running after us (ibid., p. 198).

The childlike belief that the moon is alive and is following us intention-ally (animism) is coloured by the belief that the heavens take an interest in us. Only in latency does the child learn to recognise an observation independent of herself.

One example using the subject's "brother" demonstrates how a child can either see things from another person's perspective or is trapped in egocentric thinking.

Piaget asks the five-year-old Paul, who has a brother named Stefan, whether Stefan himself has a brother. Paul answers no, with the rea-son that "there are only two people in our family. And Stefan doesn't have a brother." Paul is incapable of leaving his own point of view and observing himself from another person's vantage point—he is arrested in intellectual egocentrism, a characteristic of intuitive thinking. A child in latency can see that he has a brother Stefan and that Stefan has him as a brother, thus understanding the reciprocal function in the sense of a symmetrical reversibility.

Another example of developmental change in collective child behav-iour is revealed in their new approach to rules of playing together. Piaget gives the example of marble games. Before the latency phase, children play marbles together, where everyone knows a few rules such as how to roll the marbles, what patterns they should make, the order of the moves, etc. Nevertheless, every small child devises his own game and only cares about his own rules, not observing others or how they are playing. "In reality, each child plays in his own fashion, without any kind of coordination" (1964, p. 226). When the children are asked who has won, they are typically astonished—all of them have won, meaning only that each of them has had a good time.

Players older than seven also do not know all the rules, but they make sure to keep rules uniform during any one given game, discuss-ing them and checking them, agreeing on some rules for one game and then changing them for the next. They compare which rules are opera-tive for each of their respective games. "Winning" also has acquired a different meaning: "It means finding success in a regimented com-petition" (ibid.). The recognition that one player has won the game is based on logical discussion and acknowledgement of the rules by all participants, thus affording a new quality of common experience and a feeling for fair conduct with recourse to rules applying to all.

From impulsive behaviour to the beginnings of reflection

Instead of acting impulsively as is usual for the small child in the stage of intellectual egocentrism, the latency child now begins to reflect before acting. "Yet reflection is nothing other than an inner discussion, conducted as if it takes place either with partners in dialogue or real, outer counterparts," writes Piaget (ibid., p. 227): this means that the latency child has begun to free herself from her social and intellectual egocentrism. The beginnings of logic are based on the ability to real-ise the vantage point of other persons. "As far as emotional life is con-cerned, the same system of social and individual coordination achieves an ethics of cooperation and personal autonomy, as contrasted to intui-tive, heteronomic ethics of small children" (ibid.).

These thought processes presumably correspond to what Feldman and Ron Britton describe as the consequences of mastering the Oedipal conflict—when the child abandons the desire to banish the parent of the same sex and assume his or her position. Only when the creative paren-tal (Oedipal) dyad is internalised can two thoughts merge creatively (Feldman, 1989, p. 106).

CHAPTER THREE

Latency children in therapy

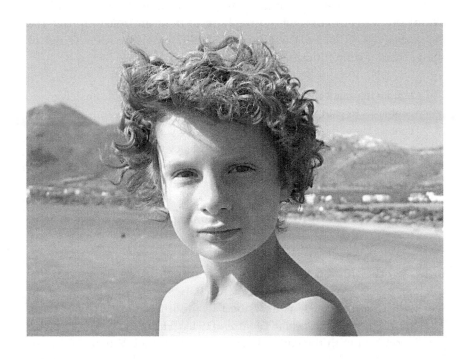

Techniques of child analysis in the latency period

I have already described some characteristics of the latency child: orientation towards learning, easy to interest, accepting of guidance. This phase of development is described as the "golden age of childhood", and is accordingly rather pleasant for teachers. Clinical experience in psychoanalysis, however, has shown that almost 70 per cent of all children who receive therapy are in this age group, most of them boys. This apparent contradiction is due on the one hand to symptomatology: learning difficulties, school problems, or the refusal to attend school are symptoms that cannot be denied or concealed. On the other hand, unconscious conflicts originate in the early years of life, when they have either gone unnoticed or been suppressed. As enjoyable as the latency period is for teachers, it is—by the same token—difficult for therapists and psychoanalysts to achieve access to the deeper layers of the child's personality, since drive impulses and sexual impulses have reached a relative standstill, with inordinately strong defence mechanisms at work.

The three pioneers of child analysis—Melanie Klein, Donald W. Winnicott, and Anna Freud—agree here in their approach. In her *The Psychoanalysis of Children* (first published 1932), Melanie Klein writes of the particular difficulties in the latency period:

> Unlike the small child whose lively imagination and acute anxiety enable us to gain an easier insight into its unconscious and make contact there, they (latency children) have a very limited imaginative life, in accordance with a strong tendency to repression which is characteristic of their age: while, in comparison with the grown-up person, their ego is still undeveloped and they neither understand that they are ill nor want to be cured, so that they have no incentive to start analysis and no encouragement to go on with it. (p. 58)

In her work with latency children, Anna Freud proposed an "introductory phase" for motivating children between seven and eleven to work with the therapist, as described in the Introduction to her book *The Psychoanalytic Treatment of Children* (1946). Here, the goal is to effect a collaboration with the child on the conscious level. When she began her career in 1927, Freud first limited her work to the latency period, but later extended her scope two years into early and middle puberty (ibid., p. 4).

> I wish to demonstrate how I succeeded in rendering the child patients (aged 6 to 11) "analyzable" in the sense of adult patients, i.e., instilling in them recognition of their illness, eliciting their trust in the analyst and analysis, and transforming the decision for analysis from an outer to an inner sphere. With this task, a period of introduction became necessary, one which is not required in adult analysis … this phase does not yet constitute true analytic work, i.e., making the patient conscious of unconscious processes, or analytic influence on the patient, does not yet occur. (ibid., pp. 14ff.)

Anna Freud characterises this "introductory phase" as "strict training" towards the eventual analysis. She means that she must first gain the child's trust on a conscious level. However, the first example given is of a small girl who says directly: "'I have a devil in me. Can he be taken out?' During the course of her three-week trial period, the little girl was then able to say that she wanted to come more often and contributed significantly to her parents' decision to put her in an extended analysis" (ibid., p. 16).

Melanie Klein conducted her first analyses with small children. With latency children as well, she attempted to first diminish the child's fears, interpreting unconscious conflicts and transference; with his anxiety relieved, the child could experience the sense and procedure of analysis. In contrast to Anna Freud's method of first exploring the conscious level of a relationship with the child without yet going into unconscious areas, Winnicott writes here of an "unconscious cooperation" (1958, p. 118). However, I find this term misleading, since through interpreting the play of the child, understanding the interconnections within her behaviour and altering her fears, it is never solely the unconscious level that is addressed—the conscious level is also present. Not only latency children but even younger children are able to explain the reason their parents wish them to enter therapy. Winnicott nevertheless writes: "In my opinion, the sooner the analyst interprets the unconscious the better, because this orientates the child towards analytic treatment, and the first relief undoubtedly gives the first indications to the child that there is something to be got out of analysis" (ibid., p. 118).

In this same article, "Child Analysis in the Latency Period", D. W. Winnicott emphasises that treating children in this age group is advisable because "... after the passing of the Oedipus complex, there develop tremendous defences" (ibid., p. 117).

What distinguishes, then, the latency child from her earlier counterpart? This distinction is predicated on the strong defence against primary-process manifestations of unconscious conflicts. Although small children express their Oedipal wishes quite clearly, in latency children these become obscured: a "successful" form of defence has established itself. Ritualised games are played again and again, and the analyst must direct special attention in order to recognise secretly held wishes and fears. One important criterion for whether an unconscious conflict has been accurately recognised is the child's reaction to the analyst's interpretation. Sometimes, the child responds with a (to the analyst) surprisingly direct "Yes", together with a deep and relieved look in his eyes. Other forms of assent could include the relief a correct interpretation elicits in the child—for instance, if during role-playing the strict teacher (played by the child) becomes a benevolent one who says that the analyst (playing the role of the pupil) has brought forth a good achievement. Or the child feels understood and consequently selects another game. If the analyst's interpretation has not shown enough understanding, the child might show criticism of it in play by (for example) making the storm his ship undergoes in the sink become a hurricane—showing the analyst that he is not merely angry at his sister's preferential treatment by their parents but indeed quite overwhelmed by stormy feelings of jealousy. Then, the analyst can put this into words and interpret: "You show me that you are not only angry at your parents and me when we give attention to another child, but that you feel threatened to be drowned by your anger like the boat. Before, I didn't understand your feelings correctly." When the play storm subsides, and the analyst receives a gentle look from the child, the child now evidently feels relieved and understood.

After several weeks of constantly playing such games, the analyst must determine how long to continue them. This can only be decided on a case by case basis, but a general guideline is that as long as access to the unconscious is made possible by a particular game, then the child should continue playing it. Even when there are no board games, cards, or iPads (as in an Anna Freud playroom) in an Anna Freud-style games room, children can bring them to therapy or construct their own out of basic materials. In therapy, the child can construct artistically creative playing cards. The central criterion is what is being expressed in (or during) play. A boy with Asperger's syndrome, after a year of successful analysis, chose the popular game "sinking ships" as a means of communication. Using table and chairs, he first built a fortress where he holed himself up, then he gave me a piece of paper and took one himself, saying that both of us should make a square with numbers and letters on it, and then draw ships of different sizes. We then took turns naming a position in order to sink the ship we had marked. Behind this apparently ritualised game, the positions from which he emerged to make contact with me afforded rich material for interpretation. Ball games where the child is more skilled than the analyst can help the analyst herself to develop new capabilities; this may perhaps change the child's behaviour from competition to generosity: perhaps he then allows the analyst to win in order to express a new spirit of friendship.

In general, the games of latency children are reality-oriented; on the one hand, fantasy is now more suppressed, and on the other hand the child's ego can take the reality principle more into consideration. Instead of showing a direct compulsion towards wetting and soiling in water games, the latency child will represent these wishes through a rationalised form of cooking and cleaning. Melanie Klein speaks of a "compulsive overemphasis on reality … since the child's ego seeks to strengthen its position by placing all of its powers at the service of suppressive tendencies, finding support in reality" (1932, p. 86). Free association, as Bornstein (1951) remarks, is experienced by the child as "a particular threat to his ego organization".

The latency child often chooses to play a role in different variations, as with Naomi, who in her school game selects the role of teacher, with the analyst playing the role of student. With role-playing, it is important to allow the child to define and describe the roles—for instance, asking the child how the analyst should behave today as student, then fulfilling these directions and only afterwards interpreting the situation as a whole. Usually, a given role-playing constellation will remain in the foreground for weeks or months until the fantasy behind it emerges and becomes comprehensible.

With other children, the central problem can already be pinpointed in the first therapy session. Winnicott describes a boy with psychotic fears, who was telling his mother as Winnicott came to bring him into his office: "But you don't understand, it's not the nightmare I'm afraid of; the trouble is that *I'm having a nightmare while I'm awake*" (1965, p. 155, emphasis in original). It is often impressive how creatively and precisely a child can express his problems.

Case studies from child therapy

I will now proceed to three case studies illustrating analytic work with latency children. The first case is given in more detail, to show how much patience is required for addressing hidden conflicts and suppressed feelings—the process Freud called "working through". Freud writes in "Remembering, Repeating and Working-Through": "One must allow the patient time to become more conversant with this resistance with which he has now become acquainted, to *work through* it, to overcome it, by continuing, in defiance of it, the analytic work according to the fundamental rule of analysis" (1914g, p. 154). Even when children's outer symptoms improve with surprising speed, careful and detailed work is required to alter the inner structures of the personality. Experiences that cannot be recalled are "activated" and expressed by the child through games. This can try an analyst's

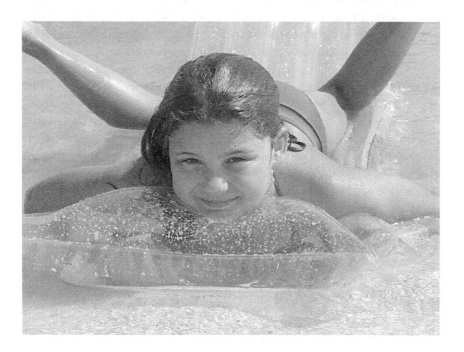

patience, as Freud pointed out. The working method of an analytic cure will now be demonstrated through the gradual shifts of Naomi's role-playing.

Girls who enter therapy tend to exhibit depressive disorders in the form of withdrawal, defeatism, and low self-esteem, or show their problems through outbreaks of rage or inappropriate behaviour. Boys are usually brought into therapy because of learning problems, fear of school, or aggressive behaviour. Now, the three case studies.

First case study: Naomi

Naomi's mother turned to me for therapeutic help for her seven-and-a-half-year-old daughter. In the first meeting, she told me that the previous year had been very difficult for everyone due to her break-up with her husband. Naomi began to eat insatiably and often had fits of rage. Her mother was concerned. One of her friends had recommended she bring Naomi to me.

Family background

Naomi is the oldest child in the family; her sister is three. Her mother was twenty-two when she had Naomi, a "wanted" child. Naomi is a vital child, full of life—but often has fits of rage, just as does her mother. The birth was spontaneous, and breastfeeding proved possible only for the first eight weeks, whereupon the mother (to her chagrin) had to bottle-feed Naomi. When Naomi was three weeks old, her father's best friend killed himself, and her father felt guilty at not having visited him the last evening he had called him. Naomi's mother was able to breast-feed her second daughter for a whole year, which made her very happy. Naomi began to speak at an early age and could already write before she started school this year.

Their marital problems caused Naomi's parents to attend partner therapy, but this proved unsuccessful. In spite of her husband's wishes to maintain the marriage, the mother decided she wanted a divorce. The father then got an inflammation of the cardiac muscle and had to have heart surgery. Naomi visited her father in intensive care (he was there for ten days), and was very worried about him. She was also allowed to visit him in rehab. The two children see their father often—as often as they wish; their mother has begun working again and very much enjoys her interesting job. The children are taken care of by a nanny, and their maternal grandmother lives in the next house. Naomi is her favourite and both children visit her often.

In the first two assessment sessions, an intensive positive transference is quickly established. Naomi is a bright child who willingly confides her feelings to me and takes up my interpretations. In the first session, she investigates the room with interest, telling me many things about her school and friends. She buries her deep fears and guilt feelings, as well as jealousy, behind exaggerated activity and manic defence; she attempts to control everyone—but not aggressively, instead flattering people in a charming and seductive way. She wants to be the only princess, and cannot admit her feelings of powerlessness and pain at her parents' separation. In countertransference, it is difficult for me (as her grandmother) to resist being blandished and seduced by Naomi and instead establish contact to her vulnerable side. Here are some scenes from the first two diagnostic sessions which caused me to recommend therapy for Naomi.

Scenes from the first two assessment aessions

Naomi arrives ten minutes late and tells me that her father was supposed to bring her but forgot the appointment.

PATIENT: (Begins to draw letters with the coloured crayons that I put on the table for her.) I already go to school and know all the letters. I hate school and would much rather be in kindergarten.

ANALYST: You ask me how it will be here with me. Will I be a strict teacher like in your school, or a nice kindergarten teacher, where you can be little?

PATIENT: I sit together with four boys in one row, I have three friends in the school—they are all girls, the rest are only boys.

She knows why she has been sent to therapy—she is eating too much and too quickly. I tell her she can come again next week and that I will then discuss with her mother whether I recommend therapy.

Interpretation

Naomi glosses over the anxiety-provoking situation with an unfamiliar woman in a new environment by precociously relating how many friends she has and her various skills. Although precocious, she tells me she would rather be small and still in kindergarten. Her statement that she hates school although she is an excellent pupil and socially well integrated points to unconscious involvement with other children and other babies. I can feel her bravely battling her stormy feelings of jealousy. In school, it is not easy to be the teacher's model student, since there are so many other children. Naomi has a young mother who could still have more children. She has successfully repulsed her mother's new boyfriend—her mother gave him up after a short time. Through her lively manner, her open eye contact, her smiling, and her conquest of me, Naomi wins my affection. Clearly, I will recommend therapy for her—she can express her problems through play and understand my interpretations.

Second assessment session

Naomi asks whether she can bring her computer game, which she has to recharge here. I interpret for her: "You don't only want to recharge your computer game here, you hope I will help you to recharge." She looks deep in my eyes and says simply, "Yes." I am fascinated by the way she can take up my interpretation.

In her computer game, she shows me how strong Super Mario can be. When I say that she would like to be just as strong, she laughs and says, "Yes, I'm the best in playing Dido and in reading." When bombs explode in the game, which fascinates her, I say to her she is showing me how she explodes when she is in a rage. She agrees and tells me how she explodes in rage when she fights with her little sister. Naomi tells of her fear of spiders and fire-spitting dragons. She expresses the wish to visit me regularly, then running quickly to the bathroom. I take up her wish later and say I will talk to her mother about the therapy; she says—as if incidentally—"I already talked to my mama, it's OK." Naomi tells how she can wrap her grandmother around her little finger. I say she is trying to do the same thing with me. She laughs and demonstrates to me how she does this: "I say, please please, dear Grandma. If that doesn't work, I pull a sad face," stretching down the corners of her mouth. "Then Grandma says yes."

Interpretation

Naomi quickly recognises that here, she can receive help; she not only feels understood by my interpretations but is also able to show this, which evokes in me as analyst a positive feeling of surprise and contact with her. It is remarkable how Naomi treats the analyst like a super-Grandma, but cannot yet show her dark side, instead emptying herself by running directly to the toilet. She presumably has great fear of looking precisely into which feelings are inside her—she wants to simply be rid of them. I can observe in her face how she empathises with every explosion in the game. Does she feel responsible for her parents' separation and her father's serious illness? Naomi is the one who decides to come back to therapy with me, and has already negotiated this with her mother. She also looks into every corner of the therapy room, wanting to take everything into her possession.

First phase—beginning of the analysis

Naomi's fits of rage point to strong unconscious tensions. She is afraid of damaging loved ones through her rage. She attempts instead to soften them up with her blandishments, just as she does here with plasticine. Her guilt feelings and aggressions against her mother's new partner indicate unresolved Oedipal conflicts and her fear of new babies.

In the session, she jumps from one game to the other, demonstrating how she jumps away from her feelings. She takes her computer game with her and is totally absorbed in it, in order to show me how she excludes me. I am meant to feel her own exclusion when her mother and father spend time together with their new partners. She conceals her helplessness, and her experience that her parents separated against her wish, by demonstrating her superiority to me; she climbs on the chair to be taller than me, and I am then the small girl who looks up to her.

Naomi talks about her daydreams. She is the only one who passes the super test in maths—all the other children fail, and she is the only one to be promoted to the next grade, with a new teacher. Subsequently, she tells me about a new girlfriend whose father has died and whose mother is sick in the hospital. If she were to get a stepfather, she would slit her throat. Then she asks anxiously: "Does it hurt, when someone dies?" She opines that it would be as simple as going to sleep. Then she corrects herself: a stepmother would be OK for her if she made really good cookies.

After a few months, the situation has changed: school is nice, but being at home is difficult. She enjoys having my undivided attention during our sessions, and becomes less controlling. For short periods, she can come in contact with her dark feelings—when she talks of her sick father's girlfriend—but then hides them behind the computer game.

In one session, she tells me first that her girlfriend called her a vampire, and then says directly thereafter:

N: I'd like so much to go to my little rabbit.

A: Rabbit? You haven't told me yet that you have a rabbit.

N: Yes, I have him since yesterday. I came home and found a note in the kitchen: Go in the woods! In our garden, we have a little woods and that's what we call the woods. So I go there and look. What do I see? A cage with two rabbits. A lady and a man.

A: A male and a female.

N: Yeah, I don't know why. I'm happy that it's a male and a female, then we'll get babies soon. (She sighs.) Yes, that'll be a lot of work, when I have to clean the stall. I'll have to get up at six in the morning, to go to school at seven. Yesterday I loved them so much.

A: You'd like to know what they do to make babies.

N: I already know. When the vagina comes to the penis.

A: To the penis? Who told you that?

N: Nobody. I read it in a book with pictures. My mama said, I shouldn't read it, but I told her: "I want to." And everything I want to I do. I read it and then I had to stay in my room for two days. (She makes a guilty face.)

A: And now you saw what the rabbits do.

N: They touched each other real close by the ears, one of them held the other's ear and they kissed. They like each other a lot. And in one minute, a baby is there.

A: You want to know how it was with you, how your papa and mama got you.

N: I know already. Vagina comes to the penis and then a kiss comes. That's it. Then you can put your ear on her stomach and hear how I snore.

A: Snore?

N: Yeah, when I'm sleeping in her stomach. My grandmother did that, but then my grandfather died, and my grandmother cried for two days.

A: You're interested in the questions of birth and death, and it's hard for you to ask. You don't want to feel like a little girl, who doesn't know about it and is afraid.

N: (Lies down, takes her cell phone out and plays a game.)

Interpretation

This conversation about sex functions as a defence: Naomi is confused, conflating the rabbits with her mother and father. I am also confused— not sure at first how much she knows about sexual union—and can empathise with how difficult it must be for her to ask. It is difficult to follow Naomi emotionally and her relative incomprehension about sexuality, an unknown that disturbs and frightens her. In a manic fashion, she seeks escape and pretends to know everything already. Her sexual theories revolve more around oral sex, kissing, and an oral-sadistic image of the vampire. She wishes to control the rabbits—an Oedipal pair—doing as she pleases. The dramatic events of recent years, her parents' separation, her father's serious illness, then both parents' new partners—all this is suppressed. Her turbulent feelings and fantasies about sexual union are split. She cannot bear all these thoughts and questions; she is more burdened that she wishes to show.

Further progress of therapy

In the following phase, she becomes the strict teacher and I am the child who refuses to do my schoolwork. She starts our first post-holiday session as if we had met the day before.

She tells me I should have done the schoolwork 100 times over. I tell her: "Once again, you are the strict teacher and I am the child. You continued this session as if there hadn't been two weeks of vacation and you were here yesterday." Naomi answers: "Yes, exactly. Maybe you have to do the schoolwork only thirty or forty times."

A: Because I understood how much you suffered from our long break, you're letting me off a lot of the work. For you, these two weeks seemed very long.

Then she commands me to do division exercises: XX divided by 1. I tell her she is showing me she does not understand her parents' separation.

N: I don't want to come to therapy at all; my grandmother gives me a present if I come to you.

Later, she sends me into the waiting room because I never complete my schoolwork the way she told me to.

Interpretation

In our role-playing, I do not turn in the schoolwork the way she wanted it done, which bothers her and makes her fearful. Naomi has a powerful superego that punishes her, just as she punishes me when I don't hand in my assignment. In role-playing, she wants me to experience how she herself feels: she is not good enough, she feels alone and excluded. She tells me she doesn't want to come to me, and I am meant to feel hurt, alone, and excluded. Perhaps she misses her mother. Bion emphasised that someone can bear loss when she has a stable, benevolent inner object, but cannot bear loss when she feels left alone with a bad inner object. I am sent into the waiting room, which signifies punishment. In role-playing, Naomi can better express important themes, a better atmosphere prevails, she does not need to jump around so wildly, and exhibits less defensive behaviour. Her portrayal of the strict teacher shows me that inside her she has a strict, harsh voice that reproaches her for being a bad girl. At the outset, however, she shows me that I am not the terrible Frau Diem, but that she is happy to be here again and to bring her problems to me.

At the next session, she hops in on one leg, because she has stubbed her other toe. With a sly smile, she hops over to her drawer, takes out the tape, and binds my hands to each other. I tell her that she is binding my hands because she does exciting things with her hands at night, even when she does not want to, and that she then wets the bed and has wild fantasies.

Interpretation

Naomi wants to prevent me from doing something forbidden with my hands. What could I do with my hands? Masturbate? Is she excited when she thinks about what her mother and father do with each other? She wants to prevent me from being active. Later, she also wants to bind my mouth, which I do not allow. Is she afraid I could take away her father? Is she jealous of my husband, with whom I spent Christmas vacation in her fantasy?

Slowly, she begins to make more space in therapy for her fantasies and feelings. She tells me of her considerable success at school and that she is the special child for her mother and grandmother. Naomi suffers from unconscious guilt feelings at being preferred in this way. Even the existence of her little sister causes her strong jealousy and quarrels. She says she hates her sister and her sister's friends because they always take her toys and break them. In therapy sessions, she shows great interest in the other children's drawers. Since she has the highest drawer, she is convinced she is the most important child for me, too.

As is typical for latency children, she always plays the same games. In this phase of therapy, her game is role-playing: Naomi is the teacher, sometimes strict, often punitive, seldom friendly, and sometimes supportive.

One scene from a therapy session after six months

N: Now we're going to learn religion. You have to answer my questions: Who was Joseph? Do you know? He was the king of Egypt. How many brothers did he have?

A: He had six siblings. You are very concerned about what happened to him because he was his father's favourite.

N: (With a strict voice.) How many siblings? Eleven! Gertraud, you're not listening: he had eleven siblings. You said it wrong. (She goes to the couch and jumps around wildly.)

A: You are very upset when you talk about Joseph. You think you are just as spoiled as he was, and then something bad will happen to you, as bad as happened to him.

N: What did they do to him?

A: You know that they threw him in a deep well, but you want me to say it and not you.

N: (Jumps around.) Be quiet, be quiet. (Gets off couch.) Come and show me what you wrote. Oh, everything is right.

A: Now you are a friendly teacher and you feel relieved because I have understood that you are afraid to experience something like Joseph did.

Interpretation

Naomi is a very gifted child, who is now learning enthusiastically in school since she could work through her great jealousy and guilt feelings in therapy, as has been shown in jealousy transference to the other children in therapy. Her mother is proud of her. Naomi is very occupied with learning and achieving; at times, I become the ignorant child. Yet when I understand her problems, I become (in the role-playing) the smart child, who answers correctly. I am meant to discuss threatening constellations for her, as if it were too dangerous for her to speak these words. She wants to have a relationship with me as with her mother; there is hardly room for a third object, for another person such as my husband. On Friday before the weekend, she feels excluded.

In this phase, Naomi is enormously possessive, she wants to have everything, see everything, investigate everything. Often she is already waiting for me at the entrance door—then she runs in front of me, and as soon as I open the door she quickly pushes me into the room, sometimes slipping between my legs in order to get into my kitchen where the door is still unlocked. Or she tries to take a look into the other children's drawers, which I have not yet locked. Full of triumph, she takes everything into her possession; she has a penetrating quality. She wants my attention so fully that I am meant to lose interest in everything else. She is like my partner, she wants to be everything for me.

N: (Again, she has run ahead, slipped into the kitchen, and discovered a game that she had taken from another child. She knows that it doesn't belong to another child now. She is bursting with pride at her cleverness.) Now I managed again to get into the kitchen. You can't work things well enough that I don't manage. Now I have not only the motorcycle that another child forgot, I also have this game. I love it. I can take it, because it doesn't belong to another child.

A: You are showing me how unbelievably important it is for you to take me and my apartment into your possession. You want everything I have to be yours. It was a long weekend without coming to me, and now you burst right in.

N: I am smart and clever, I told you that. Today is parent–teacher conference day. My mama is called for 18:30. I'm going too, and when my mother's talking, I can play in the garden with my friend, I love that … my mama will hear that I am a very good student, I always do my assignments and get a great 1A grade in German. (While she is speaking, she sticks animals and blocks onto the drawing of a farm.)

A: You are trying now to talk about how good you are at school, so that you and I forget that you just have that game … (I search for the right word.)

N: Stibitz. The game will stay in my drawer now, nobody will miss it.

A: You know it is my game, and you simply took it away from me.

N: If you hadn't left the door open, then I couldn't have got in. It's your fault.

A: You want to transfer the responsibility to me quickly.

N: Now I've played enough. (She puts the blocks back and puts the whole game in her drawer.) … Sometimes I help other children at school.

A: You help other children?

N: No, I'm the teacher's assistant and help her to monitor everything. And when I see a mistake, then I have to know what the right answer is … (She tells me how much extra work she does to get better grades.)

A: That sounds like school is fun for you. Earlier you said how much you hate school.

N: Yeah, that's changed. Now I like going to school. I'm going to take that to school too (a piece of paper with letters on it): that will be good for my grades … Today I'm going to make it comfortable here and rearrange the furniture. (She actually does begin to push the couch away, roll up the carpet, meanwhile commenting on this.) I have a very good idea for rearranging the room, you'll like it.

A: You want to be the one controlling things, as I can see. It's as if you are the owner and you're in control.

N: (She indeed manages by herself to push a small chest of drawers to the other side, the couch to the opposite wall, arranging the little table as a bedside table, the big table, and chairs on the table.) Now it looks comfortable. (She jumps around. Then she spreads the blanket on the couch and lies down there.) Now this is my room. (She shows me how she can sleep and go to the bathroom at night. She jumps around.) Life is great.

A: When you change everything the way you imagine it, and I watch you doing it, you make a comfortable room for you and me, and you and I are supposed to live here, no other child, no other husband.

N: You can't change it till I come back! (She repeats this several times with her utmost charm and powers of persuasion.)

A: You know I will put everything back after your session, but you want to convince me to leave it.

N: (She wants to rearrange the waiting room too, which I do not allow—only in the playroom. She takes her pink shoes to the coat rack.) Now it looks nice. I told you I have good taste.

Interpretation

Naomi is much freer in her playing, she is able to exhibit her intelligence and zeal for learning, pleasure in learning new things, and receives praise and gratification. She is full of ideas, can envision new interior decoration and impresses me with her truly clever and tasteful furniture arrangement. The room becomes a truly comfortable girl's room. It is meant to be an apartment for her and me: we should be enough for one another.

Concluding phase of therapy

Naomi's most frequent character in role-playing is the teacher, with me in the part of the child. She is the adult who knows everything, instead of being the ignorant child who fails to understand. The game entails a sort of development that I can observe as I myself participate. After Whitsun vacation, Naomi returns and continues her role as teacher.

N: Listen Gertraud, sit down at your desk, we'll continue where we left off. (She takes my hand and leads me to a chair where she has previously put a little table. Then she sits in my chair.)

A: You want to sit in my chair and take my place, and I should be the little child who knows so little. What kind of student am I?

N: You are a good student, you work hard to get good grades. Don't talk, do your assignments. (She sits at the teacher's desk and sorts all my assignments, marks my mistakes, and assigns plus points.)

A: You want me to be a good student, you are my teacher, and we are enough for one another, we don't need anyone else. No colleagues, no other students, no husband. We are enough for each other.

N: Right, keep on writing (with a gentle voice and crooked smile. She sees whether I need help or other writing materials, then she goes quickly off to the bathroom.) Our lessons will go on and on, there's no end, never.

A: You mean there is no interruption, no pause, and we will go on to the next session, then you don't need to be sad and won't feel any farewell.

N: Yes, exactly. You didn't make one mistake in your assignment.

Interpretation

Through play, Naomi is able to express her wish to not experience separation, to not feel grief and pain. The quality of her play has changed; she is no longer the strict teacher, but instead empathetic and supportive. Does she now have a less strict superego voice, is she better able to tolerate herself? When she comes in contact with her feelings for a short time, she runs to the toilet to excrete them, to be rid of them. She also receives much affection and attention from her parents.

Before summer vacation, her mother left a message on my answering machine saying Naomi cannot come to me in the first week after vacation, since she will be attending dance camp. After vacation, Naomi's father leaves a message on my answering machine. When I call him back, he says Naomi's mother asked him to let me know that they want to try doing without therapy. I am able to make him understand that after the traumatic experiences of her parents' separation, Naomi ought to have the chance to work through the separation from her analyst. He promises to discuss this with her mother. On Monday he calls me up again and says it would be OK for Naomi to come to a final session tomorrow. Naomi's mother calls me in the evening and informs me that now their divorce is formally completed. Naomi can come once more and say goodbye.

The closing session

Naomi is already eight minutes early; she sees the bill I have put on the table, takes it and sits down on the couch, although I have told her she should wait in the waiting room.

A: You can't wait outside today.

N: I can, but I don't want to. (Reads the bill.) This is boring.

A: Today you say it's boring, so that you don't have to feel today is a special session.

N: I know, today is the last session I come to you. Now I'm going to call up my friend J. (She goes outside and comes back for the beginning of the session. When she leaves, I feel disconsolate.) She's not at home, I don't know where she is. I don't know where L. is. I saw her at camp, but now I don't know where she is.

A: You are thinking that you won't see me again and won't know what I'm doing.

N: My mama says I don't need therapy anymore, because I don't have any fits of rage. Now I have my own room, that helps a lot. (She talks at length about her new room, and draws a plan of an apartment for her alone.)

A: While I speak of your fear about how you will do without your sessions, you draw a plan of a huge apartment, like one for a grown-up.

N: That's not true, I just made that one up. Now I have the room I shared with my sister for myself.

A: Maybe you're trying to tell me what you would do if you were big and could decide for yourself alone and could stay in therapy.

N: Yes, when I grow up, I will get an apartment. My grandma built a big building with apartments and I can choose one, and the tenant will be thrown out.

A: You're also thinking about whether a new child will come here when you aren't coming anymore. You're thinking how it is when another child comes and whether I will throw him out so that there will be room for you if you want to come back.

N: I know, but it will take a long time. Keep all my toys in the top drawer.

A: You want me to keep all your things in your drawer, and keep my thoughts about you alive in my head.

N: If it takes too long, send me my things in the mail ... Now I'm going to play a computer game.

A: What are you playing?

N: Snake.

A: The game with the snake?

N: How do you know it?

A: Was it you who told me about it?

N: (Furious.) No, I didn't! Now you have to do gymnastics as punishment! (Screams at the top of her voice.) Do five press-ups! (Approaches me threateningly.) This is gymnastics camp.

A: When you think another child told me about the game, you get furious and scream out your sorrow. Instead of thinking about it, I'm supposed to do gymnastics ...

Towards the end of the session, Naomi wants to rearrange the furniture again. When she leaves, she says, "Auf Wiedersehen, I'll see you again in four or five years."

Interpretation

After the traumatic separation from her father, and his life-threatening illness, Naomi can deal relatively well with the ending of her therapy; she attempts to take control as a defence against a feeling of powerlessness—common in children who cannot exercise control over their parents' divorce. In countertransference, I feel the psychic pain of our sudden separation, and how difficult it is for her and me to accept the abrupt end without proper notice. It is very touching when Naomi speaks of her wish that I keep her toys—which at a symbolic level must mean to keep space for her in my thoughts, a space she can retain. She knows that I will put a new child in her therapy slot. She wants me to send her her things by mail, things which symbolically express all her experiences here, everything we have played and discussed. She hopes she can come back when she grows up.

She trusts her mother's decision that she can manage without therapy, but she has mixed feelings. When she screams that I have had the game explained to me by another child, she empties herself through screaming—screaming out of herself. Instead of feeling the psychic pain and discussing it, she means it to be regimented through physical exercises. She has access to quite healthy defence mechanisms in order to deal with separation and the pain of parting, and can maintain hope that the good things she has experienced here will remain alive. She is able to recognise that she will miss the sessions, that she had a warm, safe place here, and that she had a very special relationship of trust with the therapist.

Second case study: Ben

My second case study is the eight-year-old Ben, whom I saw during my research stay at the Tavistock Clinic in London.

Referral

The school psychologist had referred Ben because he had problems with reading and concentration. The description was as follows: "He shows resistance to reading and learning new words. In maths and science, he learns better. He confuses sounds: e instead of i, a instead of e ... Ben is a bright and lovable child." Psychotherapy was recommended due to family problems.

Framework for psychotherapeutic treatment at the Tavistock Clinic

The Tavistock Clinic is part of the National Health Service; here, children and their families from a certain part of London can go for psychotherapeutic treatment covered by the NHS without charge. At the Child and Family Department, a referral is first discussed before deciding whether some kind of offer can be made for that case; subsequently, a supervising therapist is assigned to the case, who maintains regular contact with the school, the parents, and the child's therapist. In Ben's case, this supervisor was the highly experienced therapist Sheila Miller. As visiting scientist and psychoanalyst, I undertook Ben's therapy, which meant his waiting period was abbreviated, since I was working at the Tavistock Clinic for a period of one year, later extended to one and a half years. Discussions were held between Ben's parents and both therapists, during which the content of Ben's therapy was kept strictly confidential, that is, the parents were not informed.

Family background

Ben is the second child in his family; his brother Mark is eight years older. At the time of his birth, both parents were heavy drug addicts, regularly using heroin. The gynaecologist treating Ben's mother did not notice this, so that no measures were taken to detoxify him directly after his birth. Only twenty-four hours after the birth, when Ben's condition dramatically worsened, did his mother inform the doctors that she had been taking drugs up until the birth. Ben was quickly transferred to another hospital where he was detoxified. Three days later, his mother was transferred to the same hospital. For the last three years, Ben's mother has been participating in a methadone therapy programme under a doctor's control.

When Ben was three, a police raid revealed heroin at his parents' dwelling. The father assumed all culpability so that Ben's mother could remain with the children; he was subsequently sentenced to three years in prison for drug dealing, where Ben, Mark, and the mother visited him regularly. The mother is also in psychotherapy. When his therapy begins, Ben is living alone with his mother in London, whereas his brother Mark is with the father in Scotland; both father and brother are currently addicted to drugs. Ben's father has an alcoholic mother, who could not care for him adequately as a baby.

Ben's mother relates how it was mostly Mark who took care of Ben, feeding and changing him when she was not capable of this due to the influence of drugs. She says that she could not give her children regular meals, was impatient, and often yelled at them. However, she now has a new partner who establishes clear rules and makes sure they are enforced.

On the basis of all this one can presume that Ben is heavily traumatised. It will be important to centre on this trauma—which he will presumably represent through play and transference/countertransference—and help him put his experiences into words. Only then will he be able to reflect and sort out these experiences of pain and neglect. Describing all this will presumably require much patience, since Ben must have experienced such neglect, fear, insecurity, and little or no solace over the course of many years. Presumably, he has had a delayed development and has an emotional need to make up for his missed experiences. One can assume that he has lacked an understanding person, one to play with him and help him put his feelings and wishes into words, someone to read to him and sing with him. According to Ben's mother, the parents were occupied with their addiction and wild parties.

Making Ben conscious of this lack of what every child has a right to, and working through it—together with his anger against parents he also loves, and his grief over what has been withheld from him—will presumably be important themes in his therapy. It is doubtful that Ben has had an Oedipal father who could set limits. Can he learn persistence and self-confidence if he has always experienced that his drug-addicted parents turned to drugs at every frustration, instead of coping with a difficult situation? He has experienced parents who were impulsive instead of exercising patience and reflection—parents who fled into a drug-induced dream world instead of feeling psychic pain and being able to reflect on it.

Beginning of therapy

Ben first comes to me after my preliminary consultation with his mother. He is an appealing, lively child who immediately establishes eye contact with me and happily takes up the offer of therapy. At first he thought therapy would be the kind of reading training he had previously had. He is pleasantly surprised that here, he can play and we discuss it. His box of toys—which no other child can take—immediately assumes an important status. From the beginning, Ben observes me closely. He is an active boy and able to use his toys. I let him know the framework of his therapy—that he can come twice a week, that there will be a pause at Christmas and Easter, and that the therapy will last until summer.

Ben begins to draw the soldiers he has at home, soldiers who can master any difficulty. He says that he had to remind his mother that today was therapy. He asks what he should play.

A: You can play what you want to.
B: (He goes to his box and takes two tea saucers and a teapot out, pretends to make tea, pour milk and then tea in the two cups, and asks if I also want sugar, handing me one cup.) This is for you. (He takes the other cup, and we drink tea.)
A: You want to make things pleasant for both of us here, you're making tea and showing me that things should be homey for us.

B: (When we have finished drinking, he climbs on the windowsill and lets the shades down.) Now nobody can see us here.

A: You are asking me if someone is curious and wants to know what you are doing here.

B: My mother asked whether the grey wall is a board to write on. (He lets down the second shade.) Now it's night, and we're going to sleep. (He arranges the pillow, spreads out the blanket, and lies down with his upper body, his legs on the floor. Then he slides down to the floor.)

A: (I am confused and do not know what he means to express. A threatening mood seems to prevail as opposed to a happy one.) You are falling out of bed and showing me that nobody sees it.

B: (He keeps repeating the move, falling off the couch and lying on the floor, then he climbs back on the couch and falls slowly down. Subsequently, he stands up, goes with closed eyes to the sink and drinks water, and then returns.)

A: (I repeat how difficult it is to manage all this alone and how much it hurts when nobody helps him. He has to do everything alone.)

B: (Then he asks me to help him, to spread the blanket over him.) I am a very little Ben.

A: How old are you then?

B: Very little, maybe five years old. (He stands up again, walks around with closed eyes, running into furniture; then he falls down and lies on the floor.)

A: (It doesn't seem like a game, but something more threatening when he lies on the floor so lifelessly—then standing up without opening his eyes and feeling around, looking for something to drink. He seems to want to create confusion and perplexity in me, and observes me now and then.) You are showing me how it is when somebody walks around strangely, doesn't see anything, doesn't know his way around, and then lies on the ground as if he is dead. I'm supposed to be worried since I don't know what's the matter with you.

Discussion

At first, Ben shows how he feels connected to me through drinking tea, we are having an hour together, he knows he will be coming regularly and shows his link to me. Ben also took a roll of tape and taped us to one another, to show me that we should be completely together: he wants to remain the whole year with me. He takes care of me and makes tea for me, in order to show me what good it does him to care for me.

Now and then, Ben tells me that it is his responsibility to arrive punctually for our sessions. Sometimes his mother oversleeps or forgets the session. He then makes her get ready quickly—sometimes they arrive in a taxi, in order to be on time.

The sequence of falling out of bed is repeated again and again in the first weeks. In the scenario, it is sometimes morning and he has to go to work. He observes me precisely and it seems important to him to confuse and worry me. When he lies so strangely on the floor, he seems dead. Only gradually do I understand that he wants to convey to me how he felt when his parents and their friends were lying around on the floor in a drug-induced stupor, incapable of any action. He evokes this feeling in me, thus communicating something very important: this is how he felt then, and nobody understood him or talked with him about it. I describe my feelings and link them to the assumption that, as little Ben, he was very confused when his mother and father would suddenly behave in such an altered fashion. In the framework of the game, I then ask Ben what I should do. He says I should try to talk with him; but he then turns his head away and rolls over on his other side, stretching out all his limbs. I describe how disappointing it is when I would so much like to talk to him and he doesn't react, whereupon a little smile passes across his face. He cannot put his early traumatic memories into words or drawings, but he can demonstrate them and evoke them in me though a projective identification—a primitive but effective form of communication.

In one of the next sessions, as he goes to "sleep", he sticks his fingers in his eyes so that I can only see the whites, which looks gruesome. He derives satisfaction in hearing me describe how gruesome this looks and telling him I don't know what it can mean. I ask whether it could be a Halloween mask. (Ben sits up.) He says: "Now you do it!" (He demands this again and again, and I try to find out what indeed it means for him.)

Repeating the frightful, threatening scenes with his drug-addicted parents enables Ben to see them anew from the perspective of an eight year old—one who is not left alone with these scenes but now can share them with me. He also is afraid of his own feelings—feelings he has no words for. Finding words for the threatening physical and psychic conditions of his parents together with Ben enables him to sort them out and integrate them anew. He has survived these horrors.

Another theme is Ben's fear of his aggressive feelings. He comes to one session with vampire teeth that he inserts expertly into his mouth, scaring me. When I arrive at the session too late, he cuts a plasticine snake into pieces.

Ben is showing me on the one hand how I have cut off his time with me by a few minutes—but also how enraged he is at me and how he sucks my blood in his fantasy as a vampire. When I interpret this for him, he can take up my interpretation and also tells me how longingly he awaited me, and how I almost stepped into a puddle in the courtyard.

Further course of therapy

Ben develops a positive transference to me, appreciates the regularity of his sessions, and trusts our work together. He jumps from the table or windowsill onto the couch, conquering this distance. Presumably, this distance expresses the time between our sessions. I interpret this as his symbolic capacity for linking the two sessions emotionally in spite of the days that pass between them, and showing how connected he feels to me. I also understand it as an indication that he has internalised his image of me as a therapist and can keep it alive when he is not with me.

In play, Ben is able to represent the fears persecuting him: cushions become sharks that threaten to bite him, and therapy is a place where he finds refuge and security. He represents the opposite side when I become stupid and unreliable for him as do his inner objects. When I don't know an English phrase such as "out and about", I become a stupid object.

In English, my name can sound ridiculous, since "Wille" is pronounced like "willy"—a slang word for penis. Ben gives me a Christmas card and advises me of this contingency—he's embarrassed for my name, since everyone laughs when he says it out loud. I become an object of ridicule like his narcotised father, who embarrasses him, who sits in jail; he has virtually no respect for his father, since the father behaves in an unworthy and ridiculous fashion.

Ben idealises violence and negative strength, in direct opposition to his wish not to give up and to atone for wrong.

Illustration from the twenty-ninth therapy session

In the two weeks before Easter vacation, Ben begins to play a form of hide-and-seek. We take turns hiding a small soft ball somewhere in the therapy room, and the other one should search for it. In this twenty-ninth session—the last one before Easter vacation Ben once again heads straight for his toy box and takes the little ball out, looks at me smiling, thus demonstrating that he wants to play the game again. Today, he managed to get his mother to bring him to the session on time.

A: You come today to this last session before Easter on time so you can have your last session in full, and you show me that you want to play the game again, as if you were here yesterday.

B: (He laughs in agreement, throws the ball at the wall, catching it again expertly.) Now you leave.

A: (I leave the room, keeping the door a crack open as usual. This time Ben takes longer to call me back in to look for the concealed ball. I find the ball, and Ben likes this.) You are showing me how important it is to see how I leave and return, and that the ball disappears and reappears. You want to know whether you will find me back here after Easter.

B: (Does not take up my interpretation, continues to play. He then finds the ball I had concealed for him. When he subsequently conceals the ball again, I find it behind the radiator but cannot retrieve it. Ben observes precisely my various attempts to extract the ball from behind the radiator.) Give up, you won't manage. Give up.

A: You would like to see how quickly I give up in a difficult situation. Will I leave the ball in a dirty place? (I continue to try, but don't succeed.) I give up.

B: I never give up. (He forces his little hand between the tubes in the radiator, just managing to retrieve the now dirty ball.) The ball is dirty. (He goes to the sink, cleans the ball, and dries it with his own paper towels from the toilet that he has stored in his box.)

A: Sometimes I am completely incompetent, I can't take care of the ball, can't get it out, I just give up. And you show me how important it is for you and the ball not to give up and to try everything—and then you manage. You also manage to clean the ball.

B: In the vacation week, I'm going to my brother's and my father's.

A: You also want Mark and your father to give up drugs and get help, like your mother.

Interpretation

For Ben, separations are particularly disturbing; he has often experienced his parents leaving to return in a completely different state—on drugs. He wants to see if his therapist is (more) reliable. The game of looking for the ball calms him; he experiences repeatedly that both of us do indeed find the ball. He needs this calming effect and the experience of a reliable object. The game never loses interest for him, never acquires even a trace of routine. Ben brings his full concentration to the game, observing my facial expressions and movements precisely. I describe my behaviour and his to him, since he did not have a loving, understanding mother who helped him to put his feelings and wishes into words. When he cannot retrieve the ball from a hiding place, he panics. He experiences how quickly fear overcomes him, then reacting in an agitated fashion. His mother—and, in transference, I as his therapist—often becomes an unreliable, helpless person. In various ways, we re-experience and work through Ben's trauma during his sessions. Step for step, he becomes able to master it mentally and reflect on it with his therapist. As Winnicott says, therapy constitutes a "transitional space".

B: (Towards the end of one session, Ben wants me to put a pillow over my head so that I will not see. When I refuse, he puts pressure on me.) Do it. Get a move on! You're wasting our time!

A: You want me to see nothing and be helpless. I can put the pillow in front of my eyes, and then I won't see anything.

B: No, you have to put it over your whole head, just as I told you to. (He becomes quite angry and continues to put pressure on me.) What time is it, is the session over already?

A: You want to be the one who controls me, and you get angry when I don't do it. You want to be the one in control.

B: (Noisily pushes the furniture he previously rearranged back to its original position.)

A: You are not only angry because of the pillow, but it's also easier for you to leave when you're angry, then you don't have to feel how sad you are that you don't have a session next week.

B: (He looks deep in my eyes, his face relaxes, and he moves the furniture now in a calmer fashion. On the way to the waiting room, he doesn't look at me, instead going close to his mother, looking at the ground but also waving goodbye to me.)

Discussion

Ben projects his helplessness into me—I am meant to not see, to be blind; he is omnipotent and can control everything, excited by his idealisation of negative power. When upset, he quickly enters a state of hyperactivity—a mode where he no longer thinks. It is also clear that one part of Ben is glad to receive limits and experience a person who can watch over him and also protect him. Receiving clear limits is simultaneously helpful and irritating. Ben's pleasure in domination must be investigated and worked through. By the same token, it is important that he experiences his mother as reliable—that both she and the analyst return to him.

In my meeting with the parents after Easter, Ben's mother tells me that Ben is succeeding in expressing his love for his brother while also asserting his own wishes and needs. He wants to move into the bedroom of his brother, who no longer lives at home. Ben has greatly gained in self-confidence, says his mother. He observes interactions between students at school and talks to her about them. The therapy sessions are very important to him, and he makes sure that his mother gets up in time for them. The mother feels excluded, which is difficult for her. Ben tells her he is only playing in the therapy sessions and the therapist is his "friend". The mother's new partner and Ben have a close relationship. He is Ben's role model. On the one hand, Ben's mother is glad about his newly found independence, his self-confidence, and ability to reflect for himself; on the other hand, she is sad at this incipient form of separation from her—something not atypical for latency children.

He begins to more clearly express his wish to always have me by his side, as well as his irritation when I am gone over the weekend. I help him to feel this wish more clearly and to express it: "You think I contribute to your sadness when I am not there when you need me." Or: "How can I simply not be there when you feel I ought to be, then you are disappointed and irritated." He trusts himself to express anger in the sessions: on Monday, he brings balloons with him and fills them so full of water that they burst, wetting my jacket, whereupon he laughs. Ben is very relieved when I recognise his irritation over our separation at the weekend and describe it in words. He brings his warrior figures with him.

In late April, at the end of a session, Ben begins to clean out his box, parting with unessential objects. He brought stickers with his name on them and now affixes them to his ruler, his markers, his cars, and the toy gun he constructed. He remarks that now there is much more space and it is easier to get an overview. I link this to his capability for bringing order into his thoughts and now having more mental space for thinking and learning.

Discussion

Ben now has more confidence that I am less fragile than his mother when she was taking drugs. He succeeds in showing me his irritation and disappointment. In play, he shows his inner image of a stupid, unreliable mother/analyst. He can spray me with his burst balloons. Just as he can create order in his inner world and work through and integrate his trauma, he wants to make order in his box. He wants to shape the outer world in accordance with his inner world.

Concluding phase

Looking for the ball remains Ben's preferred game, but it now acquires a new intensity due to our impending separation in summer. Will Ben be able to conduct an intense relationship when it is slated to end so soon?

Often he also plays that this is his home, I am his mother and should cover him up with a blanket.

He lies on the couch and says I should cover him with the blanket and stay with him. He tosses and turns in sleep, and in the game, I ask myself out loud whether he might be having bad, frightening dreams— whereupon he increases his eye-rolling, tossing and turning. After he has forgotten breakfast in play, he switches roles: he is eighteen years old and going to college.

Then, he is my driving instructor, directing me in steering and gear-changing. He draws a picture of the gears. I pass the road test. I tell him he wants to be the one who is in control and can do everything. He is helpful and wishes to help me. He brings balls to some sessions, and explains a complicated game.

There are also sessions where he is the baby and wishes to be taken care of by me.

Discussion

Ben wants to impress me, to be the big impressive man for me. He is the one who wins. There are several clear indications of his Oedipal desires: the ball he sticks in his pants or trouser pockets. He hears from his mother how impressed she is with his growth spurt and his manly muscle development. Alternately, Ben shows his infantile side, where he wishes to make up for much of what he missed as a baby, but also the impressive eighteen year old he wishes to become. When he plays the baby, he makes only sounds and eye contact. I provide the entire dialogue myself as mother of an infant, describing his noises and movements as answers and then reacting. I feel reminded of Daniel Stern's description of a mother talking to her baby, where she allows enough pauses between what she says to him for him to answer (although he cannot yet do so in words)—in other words, she establishes the rhythm of a dialogue.

Ben and his mother learn that I have extended my stay until Christmas and that Ben can thus continue to see me. This extension of the therapy provides more time—but Ben is also encouraged in his manic fantasies of omnipotence to accomplish everything himself. He is convinced that his urgent wish to not let me go was the reason I extended my stay. He now hopes to repeat this success.

In the last month before ending therapy, Ben brings his toy figures and with them depicts various situations of separation. I describe these separations and link them to the impending separation from me. Once, Ben brings a large boat and makes it sail on the water with all his figures on deck. A storm comes, which I interpret as the storm within him since he does not want to give me up. He corrects me in play, making the storm ever wilder. I tell him he is showing me that I have not truly understood him: inside him is not only a small storm but a huge tempest, because he has such tumultuous feelings—he does not want to relinquish me and does not want to be friendly but is disappointed and deeply angry. Only when I understand his wish to stay with me forever and that I never leave him can he describe how much he misses his brother and how much he would like to go on with his life. Ben is then able to allow the mother and father figures to come together in his play. One part of him can allow me to be together with my husband in his fantasy. He appreciates the relationship his mother has with her new partner, who has undertaken a loving relationship with Ben and constitutes a reliable figure for him.

Discussion

In his therapy sessions, Ben has succeeded in expressing his feelings clearly through play—something Bion described as the "experimental self". Ben also experiences his own irritation and can reflect on it: "I am irritated," which Bion terms the "reflective self". Ben manages both modes—intense experience and distance from it, which is the basis for reflection—with the therapist's aid. It is simultaneously important to accept the Oedipal pair—both through transference, that is, me and my husband, with whom in Ben's fantasy I will reunite in Vienna, as well as his mother and her partner. In countertransference, it was not easy for me to bear Ben's aggression evoked by my impending departure or to confront myself with this aggression, instead of becoming weak and wanting to cover it up. Saying goodbye to London and my first child in therapy there was not easy emotionally, either for him or for me.

Summary

Ben's reading problem seems to centre on the fact that he cannot concentrate on letters because all his attention goes towards attempting to recognise what mood his parents (as primary objects) are in or how accessible they are. Only when he can express his own feelings, his fears, and disappointment at being neglected (mostly through projective identification onto me)—but also feel and sort out those feelings with my help—does he establish psychic space for thinking.

Like his brother, Ben is a child who early on was forced to assume the duties of an adult. He was his mother's confidant, was overtaxed by this, and lacked a sheltered childhood. Simultaneously, he possesses an almost visionary strength, he does not give up, and knows he has much of value in him. He is curious and wishes to investigate the world and his therapist—what she is thinking, feeling, what she thinks of him, whether she understands him. Is she like his mother, who so often was occupied only with herself and her own needs?

Working with Ben's mother presumably also helped her to draw clearer limits to him and try to hold to them. Through the relationship with her new partner—a warm-hearted, empathetic, and determined man—she has succeeded in stopping Ben when he hits her on her bottom or grasps for her breasts. She can feel herself as part of a pair, something that relieves Ben of a major burden. She can show her grief over the irrevocable departure of her older son Mark, thus also helping Ben to feel his grief and discuss it with her. Ben acquires all Mark's things that Mark does not wish to take along.

Ben's neglected part found a home in therapy (he stored away a large provision of paper towels). He was able to experience what it is like to express the wish of possessing me entirely. He succeeded in transforming his primitive impulses into thoughts that can be thought, as Bion has put it. His panic at making mistakes or not understanding something was lessened.

Ben identifies himself with his therapist, someone who can observe and reflect, someone who wishes to understand him and reflect on him. He manages to hold his attention and concentrate, since his unconscious conflicts and fears have become visible and discussable. In school as well, he now recognises and corrects himself when he makes a mistake in reading. He has now caught up developmentally; he has matured into an athletic, good-sized boy. He can express his need for recognition at home through play when he plays with his mother's partner—not only infantile games, but games of ball or other skills normal for a ten year old. The deprivations of his early years were successfully compensated for and worked through in therapy, supported by his improved family situation. Only when anger and sorrow over inadequate solace, love, and support are worked through can a process of healing begin.

Regular contact to Ben's school ensured a close cooperation: Ben received a new, stricter teacher, who treated him affectionately but also made sure rules were enforced. This teacher introduced a system for helping Ben to express his needs while also learning patience. He gave Ben two cards, a green and a yellow. When Ben urgently needed the teacher, he held up the yellow card; when he felt he could wait a bit, he held up the green card. This functioned excellently.

Ben's development in symbolisation and language skills was impressive. At school, he had no problems anymore—quite on the contrary, his teacher praised his creativity and the subtlety of his written exercises.

The preceding two case studies were meant to demonstrate the manifold nature of therapeutic work with latency children. Each child has a unique history, which must be investigated and treated in therapy. The third case study—Elfi—will demonstrate how a girl with subnormal intelligence can profit from child analysis.

Third case study: Elfi

Eight-year-old Elfi came to me three hours a week because of her great emotional and learning problems.[1] She was a child bereft of hope, who hid her unhappiness and desperation behind a cheerful façade, unwilling to take anything in. I see that her problems are due to early deprivation and a lack of containment. Her family situation seems good on the surface—the family is complete, her father is a successful entrepreneur, her mother stays at home with an au pair babysitter, there are two older brothers who attend the same school as Elfi. Behind the façade, however, her parents' marriage has been broken for some years. Elfi's conception was the last time her mother allowed sexual intercourse with her husband; since then, the parents live together without conducting a sexual relationship. The mother does not have a room of her own but instead sleeps on a mattress or in one of her children's beds, while one of them sleep in their father's bed. The official reason for this separation is the father's loud snoring. Snoring is an attribute of the father's body—which the mother avoids. As becomes clear in the parent meeting, the father would be interested in a full sexual marital relationship, but does not want to be rejected. Everything remains in a diffuse half-light.

Excerpt from an analysis session

Elfi's mother informed me at the beginning of the session that she was going to have a small operation and that Elfi would be brought to the session the following week by the au pair girl.

Elfi plays the same game with little wooden figures as in the previous session: she takes the pink girl with a little sister, and I must take the bad, blue figure. She shows me how beautifully she can fly, demonstrating these movements. The other wood figures are also wonderful fliers—only I can't do this, with my blue figure. Elfi and the other animals want to kidnap me. I must be very, very fearful. I keep expressing how frightened I am and how well she can do things, how badly I do things. She says I should only watch now, and put my figure on the table.

I interpret that she wants me to be the fearful little person who can't do anything. She is the big strong person, who can fly and is listened to by everybody, and who tells us what to do.

E: Yeah, look what I can do! (She flies artistic loops with her figure, steep ascents and crashes.) Now you should be afraid and fall off the table.

A: (I bring my figure to the table's edge and make it look down.) Now I am afraid to fall off. You want me to feel what it's like when I am afraid, when everything falls apart.

E: (Laughs loudly, takes my figure between two fingers and puts it in the middle of the room.) Here everything is full of water. First only a little, but it's getting higher and higher and you get more and more afraid, because you can't swim. You should be more afraid.

A: There is so much water, it's getting more and more and I don't know what I should do. I'm so afraid.

E: (The situation becomes ever more dramatic, and I am meant to express my fear ever more intensely.) Now sharks are coming, one two three of them, they are hungry and want to … (she breaks off).

A: You are showing me what it is like to be more and more afraid, not to know what the results will be of your mother's medical examinations. You think it is very dangerous.

Elfi tries to hold my mouth closed and says: "Please, don't talk." She goes to the couch and says: "I'm bored."

She has great fear of admitting her concern over her mother, her fear of losing her. This fear becomes more and more clear in her play—but as soon as she is connected to the cause of this fear, she interrupts the game and becomes bored, since she cannot admit to the feelings that are actually relevant. She wants to hide all her wooden animals as she hides her feelings. I am meant to close my eyes. When her mother comes to pick her up, she doesn't want to leave. I am meant to leave everything the way it is. Elfi goes to the buzzer and presses it to let her mother in.

In the next session, she hides and I am meant to look for her; she hides under the table, covering herself with a blanket.

A: You would like me to look for you and you are showing me that you want to hide yourself and your feelings.

E: (She looks for me, then saying:) You are a doll. (She takes me by the hand and leads me, since she says I cannot walk by myself.) You have to make very small steps, like a doll.

A: Now you are the one who can walk and control things, and I am the doll and should do what you want.

E: (She feeds me with a wooden block.) You are hungry, tell me whether you want more to eat.

A: I'm so hungry, I want more to eat.

E: Now it's enough, because you can't go to the bathroom.

A: You think I should eat more and more, until I have a fat stomach.

E: (Changes her mind and leads me to the bathroom, reassuring me that it will only be in play. She puts the toilet seat down and lets me sit on it. Then she leaves and says I should cry, since I'm so afraid.) You are crying and crying, but nobody hears you. (When she then turns the light on, the fan goes on too, and she tells me as the doll what that is. Then she takes me again by the hand, prepares a bed for me and puts me to bed.)

A: You are the person who is in control and I should feel how it is to be afraid and be all alone. You are showing me how much fear you have and that nobody wants to know about that, nobody listens to you.

E: Don't talk, you are a doll and can't talk or understand anything. The bed is unfortunately hard, but that's how it is. (She tells me that I should ask her when she is coming back.)

A: When are you coming back?

E: You belong to me, but if you don't behave yourself, I'll send you to another child, my neighbour, who visits me every day. (Since I was bad while she was putting me to bed, she calls up her friend, talking with her like an adult, and telling her she will send her a doll.)

Interpretation

Elfi shows me how her mother makes her into a doll and how dangerous it is to have feelings or the desire to live. Playing the mother, she says how hard the bed is and how hard life is. Elfi's mother herself is devoid of life, and she wants Elfi to be a good doll who cannot think or feel. Elfi is convinced that nobody listens to her and that nobody wishes to understand her. Everyone pretends to love her, but she knows she is unwanted. She, too, is left in the dark—just as I am on the toilet in her game. Does she perhaps have bad dreams at night?

Elfi feels she is an unwanted child and has great fear of losing her mother if she does not play the part of a pretty, sweet doll. She knows that the friendly countenance of her parents does not correspond to reality. Nobody wants to see her fear and despair. Nobody is able to hear how difficult life is for her. She is afraid of life, her feelings, and her sexuality. She denies her body, playing the part of the pig in our games. Nobody talks about her problems, she is left in the dark. She wants to be lifeless like a doll, to feel nothing, and identifies with her depressed, innerly moribund mother. She can dance and sing, and often plays the clown in order to cheer her mother up. She is afraid of her feelings and her vitality—her only companion is her dog, whom she loses after four years of analysis.

She exhibits massive defence mechanisms and inhibitions towards the deeply disturbed environment created by her family. Her mother cannot find a way out of her secret depression, deep pessimism, and confusion.

Behind the façade of a cheerful, stupid girl, there is rage and the hope that I can be a companion to her in her loneliness and deep desperation. She wants to find out whether I see the truth or—like her mother—console her away from it, pacify her. Often I am overcome by deep doubts as to whether I can help her, and believe myself to have completely failed as analyst—can I ethically accept the fact that I am paid to play with her if I cannot help her? Only when I sat down and wrote these feelings down did I realise that this is an exact description of Elfi's emotional situation: she feels that she is unwanted and a failure, different from the other children (and in actual fact, her intelligence is subnormal). She is convinced that nobody wants to be with her, that she is boring. Instead of acting out this scenario with her, I use my feelings for interpretations.

Indeed, Elfi does have a difficult situation in her private school—where she is the worst-achieving student. At the beginning, she was basically an outsider, and the other children teased and mocked her. When she came into analysis, she could not speak a full sentence, in fact did not speak much at all and with faulty grammar, and was inordinately fearful.

Elfi attempts to keep herself and others in the dark; everything is meant to remain vague:

E: (She comes and says with a smile:) I have to go to the bathroom badly. (Looks at me urgently.) Do you believe me? Sometimes I say I have to go to the bathroom when I don't really have to.

A: You are observing me and what I say. Whether I am confused or know what you mean. You show me that you deliberately confuse other people.

Elfi knows that her parents do not tell her the truth, and she herself tells stories. She wants to find out whether I see the difference, whether something is true or not. Elfi attempts to turn everything into a game, in order to not take her own fear and questions seriously. She builds up a massive defence against exhibiting her threatening feelings. She hopes that I at least recognise that she often deludes people intentionally. When she has to tell some story in school she has not understood, she invents one. The children then laugh. She herself knows that she is not as smart as the other children and cannot remember stories.

E: (Almost nine years old, takes a letter from her schoolbag and asks me to read it to her.) What is that?

A: You can read it yourself.

E: No, I can't read or write. Well, I can only write very, very slowly, but we haven't learned to read yet.

A: Would you like to try?

E: No.

A: (I slowly read the second line, which is her name.)

E: (Pained and annoyed.) I can't read!

A: You show me how much it hurts not to be able to read it, and that's why you don't even try. You'd like me to read it instead of you.

Elfi puts me under pressure to read both lines. She forces me to understand how horrible it is to be different from the other children, who can already read fluently: this makes her furious and helpless. When I read, she falls into despair and self-anger at her inability. She tells me that when she is eighteen, she plans to jump off the roof, since at the age of eighteen she can do what she wants. She already has jumped out the window into the garden—nobody knows of this, and she did not hurt herself. It is as if she is forbidden to employ her reason. In play, I am the stupid one, who can neither jump nor write. Only after she has experienced that she can share her desperation with me does a wish in her awake to change herself, to have a reasoning faculty with which she can think.

A: What's the matter, why are you sad?
E: If I have a wig with long curly hair and never wash it, would it grow onto my head?
A: You would like to be different, maybe to have the kind of hair I have (I have long, blonde hair).
E: I want to dye my hair, not like yours, just blonde streaks. Are you listening to me?
A: You want to be a different girl, because you think nobody loves you the way you are. You want to have not only my hair but my mind, to be able to think and do calculations.
E: I asked mama and papa, but they won't let me.
A: You hope I can help you to change something, so that you can think better.

Slowly, Elfi becomes able to admit her feelings and her despair instead of playing the clown and letting herself be treated as a doll. She convinces her mother that she can come alone to analysis. This gives her great self-confidence that she can travel by public transport to me after school. She has shed her fear of reading and—with the help of a tutor— slowly manages to learn reading and maths equations. When she has difficulties, she easily slips into a hysterical, manic mode which makes everyone laugh.

Only in the second year of analysis does it become dramatically evident that Elfi not only has massive emotional problems and intellectual inhibitions, but also is of subnormal intelligence. Her parents have her take a psychological test. For me as her analyst, it is also painful to acknowledge the reality that I cannot enable Elfi to reach a satisfactory level of learning by working through her inner conflicts and fears. With other small children I have treated analytically, their problems have turned out to be "pseudo-stupidity"; in reality, they were highly intelligent and could develop their capabilities after we worked through their fears. I would have been so happy to see Elfi take such a path. I did not want to acknowledge my handicap as an analyst: that I was incapable of conceding how handicapped my patient actually was. Waves of the same hopelessness as Elfi's inundate me, and I ask myself whether I can help Elfi at all, whether I can make headway against such massive defences and manic behaviour. I must limit my own ambition for success in my analytic work with children and set realistic aims. Elfi is a child living in an extremely unfavourable family situation, which hinders analytic work. Her mother is radically against analysis, laughing at it and characterising it as senseless and expensive. She herself lives through massive projections onto Elfi and does not actually wish any changes in her daughter. In this fashion, she manages to take care of Elfi, who is handicapped and the family failure. Can I be satisfied with a modest success, helping Elfi to develop the few abilities she possesses? It seemed to me unjust that the talents in Elfi's family are distributed in such a lopsided way. Elfi's brother is practically a genius. He was also tested for learning disabilities—but he has a supernormal intelligence and was put in an excellent private school, where he became an outstanding student. I too kept doubting my capabilities as an analyst. Was I good enough to help Elfi? At times, I discussed my work with colleagues, which strengthened my confidence in my own capabilities.

Not infrequently, Elfi surprised me with her realistic view of her own limitations. She also began to be the only one in the family to recognise her limits and identify family problems. She asked her father directly whether he loved her mother at all. The father—who did not trust himself to tell his own wife that he had been in analysis for many years—was very impressed by Elfi's frankness.

A major developmental step forward then occurred when Elfi became able to also show me her feelings of anger. I had cancelled one session, but neither she nor her mother had remembered this. She had arrived in vain, and stood before a closed door. The next day, she came to me with wet socks and lay down on the couch.

E: … Yesterday, I also had wet socks.

A: Yesterday there was no session, and you felt left alone and got wet feet.

E: (Takes the box with wooden animals and throws the lid at my head.)

A: You trust yourself to show me how angry you were and are. You throw the lid at my head because you think I threw both your hours away.

E: (Takes the green wooden girl and throws it behind her chair.)

A: You are very, very angry at me, and think I didn't want you because I wasn't here. You think I deserve it, because I didn't warn you, that's why you're attacking me.

E: She (the wooden girl) is grown up, she can live alone for a while. (She takes the pink girl, tells me it has a lot of money and can buy all the animals she wants to. She says there are ugly and beautiful animals …)

Elfi can recognise her feelings and show them in play. When I do not understand how annoyed she is at me, she throws all her wooden figures away. Only when I have put her deep anger and abandonment into words can she put herself as the pink girl into a position of power.

In transference, Elfi also shows her mistrust; she only dares to place herself in my trust briefly. Although she seems gentle, she is internally hard, masculine, and cruel. Any change can only proceed against her massive defences. Her family is not happy and not a pleasant place for her to be. Her fantasy of parental union is that the parents attack one another.

Outdoors, Elfi observes birds attacking each other with their beaks. When I wear a white sweater, Elfi threatens to make it dirty with her fountain pen. She manages to make a blue spot on it, in spite of my vigilance, which pleases her greatly. She acts as if I were responsible for this.

Her sadistic fantasies concerning her parents' sexual intercourse are revealed through the birds' fighting. She uses her fountain pen as a weapon to ruin my white sweater and breast; she wishes to attack the mother/analyst and derives sadistic pleasure from this. I am meant to feel incapable and think I have done something wrong—which I indeed actually feel, reminding myself that Betty Joseph recommended wearing a work apron during child analysis in order to be less vulnerable to attack. When I defend myself, Elfi mocks me and I become a little, fearful baby who is afraid of a fountain pen. Elfi reacts with magical fantasies of omnipotence when she is incapable of doing something: she invents stories instead of putting letters together. At home, she has no structure that helps her to put parts of herself together. Often, Elfi manages to put me in a helpless position. It is important to show her that she is angry about the analyst's vacation and for this reason wishes to do something mean, putting me in a defenceless position. But speaking clearly about this situation constitutes a new model for her—speaking the truth even when it is unpleasant or painful. She is also shocked at her own aggressive impulses.

On the technical level, Elfi's great need for control is difficult to deal with. It is essential to find a balance between clarity and sufficient flexibility, in order not to be enveloped into a conflict. When she feels small, she wants to control me (and her mother). Everybody calls her a baby, but she isn't a baby anymore—as she remarks in her second session. It is important not to be intimidated by her and not be seduced into covering up cruelty with seeming friendliness, maintaining an illusion of a friendly family/analyst. The analytic attitude is: can you bear the truth, even when it is painful or shameful? Only then is it possible to develop existing capacities instead of investing one's entire energy in suppression.

In the parent meeting after two years, the parents report that Elfi is now learning better at school, although she is very slow. Her speaking is much improved. Nevertheless, her father has to defend the analysis, which both Elfi's mother and her teacher find unnecessary. The mother proudly reports that Elfi has now read a book all by herself, taking it in her own hands. She is no longer the worst pupil and is tutored three times a week. The changes in the outer world are positive, whereas in analysis, the full extent of Elfi's disorder is only beginning to emerge. The parents decide to continue Elfi in analysis. My next book concerns puberty for boys and girls, and Elfi's development during puberty will also be discussed.

Note

1. Material from this analysis is also used in my presentation "On Techniques of Child Analysis: Supportive Interpretations Versus Containment", in the annual Vienna lecture programme, Sigmund-Freud-Vorlesungen 2012.

CHAPTER FOUR

The significance of reading in the latency period

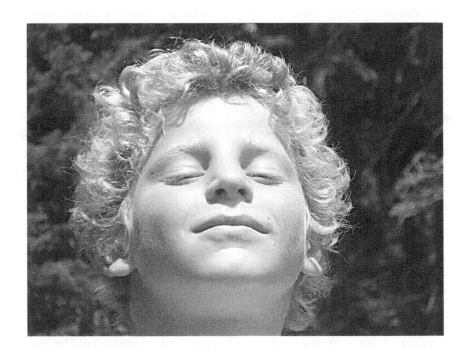

Children do not read primarily in order to acquire knowledge. Psychoanalysis theory holds thats the only texts that interest children are those that help them to express their basic emotional conflicts and satisfy their unconscious desires and hopes, thus alleviating their unconscious fears. Through reading, the child achieves a symbolic identification with the characters in the story, who solve their problems in place of the reader and master outer (and inner) dangers. In early childhood, archaic conflicts and desires are satisfied symbolically through fairy tales; sadistic or cannibalistic impulses can be delegated through identification with a dangerous, evil stepmother or dragon, a monster or bad fairy. While role-playing in therapy, for instance, a child may decide to play the evil stepmother who kills Sleeping Beauty with the poisonous apple, and the therapist should play Sleeping Beauty—in this way, the child shows her jealousy and envy of a newborn sibling, whom she would rather have dead than alive. Children thus constantly want the same fairy tales to be read to them: they already know the end of the story and can repeatedly work through their fears without anyone being actually hurt (see Bettelheim, 1976). A major difference in latency is that children can now read themselves, and are not dependent on adults (parents) to read to them.

In the latency period, reading acquires a major significance, since— as Freud wrote in 1911—children use fantasy as a defence against libidinous desires. Sexual and aggressive desires can be integrated and diverted into jokes and rhymes, similar to rubber-ring jumping for girls (Gardner & Moriarty, 1968; Goldings, 1974). Especially for small children, fantasy is expressed mostly through play, where a scene is represented through dolls or playmates. In latency, fantasy largely loses its link to physical motion (see Klinger, 1971), and can be expressed through the reading of stories, where the child identifies with the heroes of the story, who usually master dangers without parents or in a group of peers, also making discoveries or uncovering wrongdoing as detectives. Thus various forms of defence and control are formed through verbal representation—whereby neurological and cognitive developments play a major role. G. J. Donnellan (1980) believes that the development of the capacity to symbolise facilitates the child's interest in reading.

Latency children differ in their emotional needs and conflicts. This is mirrored in the various books written for them: repression of Oedipal desires and the wish for relative independence and autonomy are reflected in heroes/heroines who are orphans or whose parents are far away, so that the protagonists can and must master their challenges without parental help. Fenichel (1943) pointed out that such texts "pose high demands on the ego ideal".

Passionate reading serves as a substitute for masturbation, which is (unconsciously) why teachers may chide children for reading hours on end. Children can be fascinated by one book, unable to stop, compelled to read to the end—indications of a strong libidinal aspect to reading. Often, insatiable readers are urged to go outdoors and do sports—an analogy to preventing masturbation in the young years. Kate Friedländer recommends providing children with interesting books, that is, those corresponding to their emotional needs, and also taking the books' artistic merits into consideration (quoted in Fenichel, 1943, p. 589). When children have outgrown their latency phase, they often look back in scorn on the literature they loved during it. When reading is unable to serve as an equivalent to masturbation, a child will have trouble concentrating.

As an introduction to the child's feelings at the beginning of latency, with her emotional leave-taking of early childhood, the poem *Now We Are Six* by A. A. Milne (1927) should serve well:

> The End
>
> When I was One,
> I had just begun.
>
> When I was Two,
> I was nearly new.
>
> When I was Three,
> I was hardly Me.
>
> When I was Four,
> I was not much more.
>
> When I was Five,
> I was just alive.
>
> But now I am Six, I'm as clever as clever.
> So I think I'll be six now for ever and ever.

In fact, a child experiences becoming six as if he has now acquired an independent life. He wishes to forget his entire past, as if a new era were beginning—as free as possible from the turbulence of early childhood. However, this chance for liberation and attendant (fantasised) independence from the parents is only relative. Through attending school, the child is introduced to new authority figures, starting to place them on the same level with her parents; other children and their ways also become interesting, but the family remains the emotional nest. This transitional space between family and the social world of school and after-school activities constitutes a chance—often overlooked by parents—for affording children the experience of an independent ego. The daily separation from the family though attending school, as well as returning home each day, constitutes an important experience. Reading books enables the child to identify with a leading character, who accomplishes (in the reader's stead) those dangerous actions and developmental steps that are emotionally important—with the reader accompanying him mentally.

In this chapter, we will open a psychoanalytic perspective on children's literature, showing the themes from unconscious fantasies, desires, and emotional needs it expresses.

In the texts discussed, only peer relationships are described; the greater emotional distance to parents is demonstrated in that they are usually only present at the beginning or the end of the book. This constitutes a form of splitting which renders experiences simpler and excludes many themes.

Moral questions are dealt with in terms of good and evil in order to supply unambiguous answers. William Golding's novel *Lord of the Flies* explores such moral questions.

Collective identification is expressed through a clear "we", defining ethnic group, social class, gender, or neighbourhood. In the literature examined, authors have attempted to depict the experience of minorities—for instance, *The True Diary of a Red Indian*, which tells the hopeless story of a boy's life on an Indian reservation and his successful break into artistic independence.

Children themselves tend not to feel the unpleasant sensations of being worthless or bad, but instead project them onto other persons, such as villains who are successfully pursued and captured in detective stories. Detective stories centre on the solving of riddles, pursuing and punishing wrongdoers, as in Erich Kästner's *Emil and the Detectives* or *Lottie and Lisa*.

The desire for independence is thematised in stories of children without parents. Whether the parents are dead or simply absent, as in *Pippi Longstocking*, life must be mastered without them. Children are kidnapped or abandoned and manage to nevertheless prevail (for instance in Dickens or Stevenson). In his *Chronicles of Narnia*, C. S. Lewis sensitively explores the defence mechanisms of children who feel themselves abandoned and must prevail in an alien fantasy world.

Exploring new realms—an island where the protagonist lands, underground caves, etc.—stands for the exploration and development of the reader's self; self-exploration and knowledge in new life situations and dangers, and learning to overcome depressing, hopeless conditions is addressed in (for example) Stevenson's *Treasure Island*.

Language is a vital element and often occurs in dialogue, similar to how children use language creatively, experimenting with new words and expressions.

In hopeless and threatening situations, the settler's boy in *The True Diary of a Red Indian* does not give up—for instance, when he must survive the winter alone in a cabin in the American wilderness. He receives unexpected help from an Indian boy and his parents. In this way, the apparent advantage of the white settler is relativised, with the forgotten Indian knowledge in North America described vividly as the boy's salvation. Thus the child reader's trust in her own capacity for developing new abilities is encouraged, as well as her trust in receiving and accepting unexpected help.

In their book *Narratives of Love and Loss. Studies in Modern Children's Fiction*, Margaret and Michael Rustin name the essential criteria for a rich, high-quality children's literature in the latency phase: "One way in which these writers explore children's inner experience—we might say their relation to the figures of their internal world or to the internal objects of psychoanalytical theory—is by describing the meaning for the child of feeling contained and understood in symbolic terms" (2001, p. 11).

One important element is the capability to think, retaining an inner resistance in the face of temporary difficulties—which is made possible by the recollection of good experiences. The working through of these difficulties occurs through play, imagination, and language.

Children's literature uses such tools, also representing these difficulties symbolically through the protagonists' own development.

The potential openness of children in this age group to their own inner world makes them "good readers"—in other words, impressionable. They can be deeply moved by good stories. In contrast to fairy tales, stories for latency children are less dramatic and archaic, and almost always have a happy ending.

Harry Potter

Internationally, the most successful children's books of the twentieth century were Rowling's *Harry Potter* novels. Even children who rarely read "gobble up" these thick books. Rowling succeeded in tapping into a tradition of fantasy stories, adding elements from other genres as well as electronic media, so that the reader can simultaneously imagine "special effects" as at the movies. Rowling creates a fantastical world full of unique rules, games, and environments. Albus Dumbledore's remark concluding the first book, *Harry Potter and the Philosopher's Stone*, applies to the entire series: "My brain surprises even me sometimes" (1997, p. 217). The Hogwarts students' photos can actively wave, like electronic animation on a computer. The central game, "Quidditch", masterfully transfers the fascination of fast-moving skateboards, bicycles, or skis to witches' broomsticks. The experiences children have of switching from the real world into the virtual world of computer games, of tweeting or sending selfies, thus bridging huge distances within seconds, have a match in the magical world of Harry Potter. The fascination of modern communication techniques is here made tangible through these forms of magic, thus stimulating the great interest latency children have for extraordinary objects, fables, and arcane skills. These two worlds—the real one inhabited by Muggles (those born without magical skills), and the magic world—exist simultaneously, with an entire ministry dedicated to hiding the existence of magicians from the Muggles. At the beginning of the school year, and at the beginning of each new volume, the transition from the real world into the magic world is depicted through boarding a certain train. On platform 9¾ at Kings Cross Station, the children cross a barrier if there is no Muggle paying attention—thus embodying the reader's wish to belong to something special or exotic. Harry is the fatherless child, made to grow up in a cupboard under the stairs at his terrible relatives' with their repulsive son Dudley. Like most middle-class boys in England, he attends secondary school—but a special one, where the magician's craft is taught. Transferring to middle school is exciting and unnerving for all ten to eleven year olds. When Harry hears whispers of his impending important birthday, "... he stopped dead. Fear flooded him."

Hogwarts is a boarding school promoting imagination and understanding as central values—like an alternative culture to the boring, grey world of normal people. This boarding school binds tradition to progressive elements: on the one hand, teachers emphasise tradition and historical rituals, but on the other hand it is co-educational and ethnically mixed. The protagonists have imaginative and witty names: Professor Snape, who can also be unpleasant and envious, attends to the students' safety—his first name is Severus. First names are reminiscent of Greek myths—Minerva McGonagall—and there are also gothic, Wagnerian names such as Lord Voldemort (see Rustin & Rustin, 2001, p. 269).

Harry is a special child, a child who has even survived the murderous attacks of the powerful magician Voldemort. But this special quality only gradually reveals itself. At the beginning, Harry Potter is a male Cinderella, who grows up with foster parents, the Dursleys, and is treated badly. He has lost both parents. Only in the further course of the narrative do Harry and the reader learn that his true parents were famous and well-loved magicians. This story thus has the same point of departure as does what Freud (1909c) termed the "family romance"— the longing for a special family. At first, Harry lives in the horrid, normal world of the Dursleys and is treated badly there. He receives inferior food, has to live in a closet under the stairs, and is never treated on the same footing as their biological son Dudley. The world is depicted as black and white: in a child's imagination, there is only good and evil, victim or torturer, and heroic salvation.

Young readers find themselves in the same situation: they are searching for new authorities such as admired teachers, stars, and singers—whom they worship from afar, collecting their pictures and reading every detail of their lives in magazines. They attempt to distance themselves from their parents and join together in peer groups.

Harry Potter develops from an abject Cinderella into a hero. Zwettler-Otte points out that young readers can derive hope from this: even when their capabilities and talents have not yet been discovered, it still could be that they—like Harry—are "great, talented and infinitely loveable creatures" (2002, p. 160). In a schoolboy fashion, the magician apprentice Harry has to learn magic incantations and rules. In especially dangerous situations, memories of his parents, particularly his mother, stir in Harry. His physical capabilities, in competitive sports, are admired by girls and by his friend Ron. We see his fear of death through his nightmares after the Quidditch match, as well as his guilt feelings that he did not save his mother from her death.

Harry's emotional discovery of moral possibilities demonstrates his development and the insight that he must deal not only with outer but with inner good and evil aspects of life. Harry not only discovers his own capacity for acting on his convictions, but he also uses his intelligence and courage, supported by his two friends, Ron and the ambitious Hermione. The three of them form an alliance that can conquer dangers only when they keep together and encourage one another. Harry's maturing process signifies the capacity for integrating good and bad aspects within himself and others: he recognises that the feared teacher Snape indeed hates him, but has nevertheless protected him.

Harry's ability to perform magic takes up the magical thinking of early childhood, when children believe they actually influence their parents and the real world with their fantasies. They are convinced that an evil person can truly make someone sick or kill them, that the sun and moon rise only for them. But instead of accepting reality and relinquishing the idea of his own power, Harry goes in the opposite direction: he nurtures his ability to make magic with all the available arts and a thousand-year-old tradition. There is indeed a school for this, but it has limits and rules. This makes it all the more fun when Harry disobeys the ban on making magic in the world of the Muggles. Harry and the reader are surprised when the glass windows vanish from the zoo, fulfilling one of his secret wishes, or when his hair grows instantaneously.

Through identifying with Harry, it becomes possible for the reader to slowly become conscious of his own good and dark sides. In his holidays, Harry resolves to be tortured by his stepbrother no more, instead defending himself. Even though he is not allowed to work magic during the holidays, he can still make his stepbrother believe he is capable of doing so, thus intimidating and scaring him. Since Harry himself had to endure such humiliation earlier, the readers can now also experience relief with him. Harry also has the gumption to speak the name of his parents' enemy, Voldemort, thus demonstrating courage. His magic tricks are often like an uncovering of unconscious desires: the magic wand is not sought by the children, but instead the child is sought by the wand. The magic mirror shows Harry his deepest, most desperate wishes.

Harry is nevertheless very vulnerable; he receives a present from his father, kept for him after the father's death: the magic cloak that makes him invisible—like a protective father who takes care of his son and keeps him out of danger. Harry learns how important it is to use his intelligence and abilities not only to solve his own problems, but also to help his friends. He begins to see the world no longer in black and white opposites, but in a more differentiated fashion. He has parents who chose to die in order to benefit him and future generations. Harry lives, and he is conscious both of his limits and of the meaning of death; in this, he constitutes a role model for the reader.

The Chronicles of Narnia

As a second example of meaningful literature for latency children, I would like to discuss C. S. Lewis's *Chronicles of Narnia*, which were also adapted for film and have attained great international importance.

The *Chronicles* are a series of seven volumes, at first not planned as a contiguous narrative; for this reason there are questions between various publishers as to which should be the first volume. The first volume to actually appear, in 1950, was *The Lion, the Witch and the Wardrobe*. The title points to a crossing over from our world into the magical world of Narnia, through a mysterious wardrobe that provides passage into this secret realm. In World War II, the siblings Peter, Susan, Edmund, and Lucy Pevensie from the London district of Finchley have found protection from the Blitz through Professor Digory Kirke, and discover by chance the wardrobe: the way to Narnia.

This beginning—typically for children's books—consists in a separation from the parents, with the children now left to their own devices. The four siblings remain together and represent quite different types: the older brother, Peter, wishes to explore the world, and feels responsible for his other siblings; Susan, the older sister, functions almost as a replacement mother, taking care of the little ones; Edmund, the second brother, is ambitious and in the shadow of his older brother, whom he envies and would like to outdo. The youngest is Lucy, fearful and shy—she is the book's real heroine. Professor Kirke's large house is intimidating, and the housekeeper runs a tight ship; she does not want to be bothered by the children when she leads visitors on tours. While the children are playing hide-and-seek, Lucy discovers the wardrobe, hung with soft fur coats. Little Lucy, who misses her mother more than do the others, cuddles in the soft coats, like a substitute for the warmth and protection of her mother.

Making the youngest child into the book's heroine helps latency children to identify with Lucy. The world a schoolchild is now exploring, too, is simultaneously exciting and strange. There are new rules and modes of behaviour—so much a child cannot yet understand. The child can make words out of letters, but the meaning of many words is unknown. Older siblings and adults seem to have access to some secret knowledge that is only accessible in small doses for the younger child. Often it is difficult even to formulate the right questions without appearing foolish: Gerlinde, a ten-year-old (Austrian) patient of mine, told me she had not understood why her older sister and mother looked at the label on bolts of cloth and said "Made in England". She had no idea that this was in English. When she asked what it meant, they only replied briefly that the cloth was made in England. When she got a chance, she read out loud (phonetically in German) "Made in England"; she knew that in German, the word *"Made"* means maggot, and therefore thought the words must mean "The Maggot in England". Wishing to solve this conundrum, she only reaped scornful laughter; "Ha, ha, Gerlinde reads it as if it means the maggot in England". Telling her that it was English hardly helped Gerlinde, since she believed "English" was merely a code language, where for instance letters might be displaced. Nobody had told her how to translate words from German to English.

Our heroine, Lucy, is confused by her many new impressions in Narnia. She is dubbed "daughter of Eve" by the faun Tumnus, instead of her real name. She places her trust in this faun until he confesses that he is acting in the service of the white witch, who has instructed him to catch the sons or daughters of Eve and bring them back to her. He serves Lucy a formal English tea, playing a melody on his strange flute that makes her at once laugh and cry; she feels like simultaneously sleeping and dancing. In reality, the faun has only pretended he wishes to help her, hoping to capture her as soon as she falls asleep. But if he does not manage this, he will be cruelly punished: his tail will be cut off, his horns sawn off, and his little hooves turned into horses' hooves—or he might even be turned into a stone. Now, since he has come to like Lucy, he protects her instead and will not deliver her up to the white witch. He brings her safely back to the lantern, the portal to the human world, requesting a token from her—her handkerchief.

This initial excursion into an unknown, magic world brings Lucy's encounter with deception and betrayal to a head. Here, the book addresses how children see through the contradictory behaviour of adults who follow completely different schemes than parents. Lucy has now given the faun something of her own—a transitional object like the blankets or stuffed animals of small children, representing their mother—half symbol, half objectified. While the faun played his melody, Lucy could observe contradictory impulses and feelings in herself. These stand for "Lucy's capacity for being internally alive to her own complexity and ambivalence (…) the source of her position as heroine" (Rustin & Rustin, 2001, p. 42). When the faun becomes fearful, Lucy is able to retain her relationship to a good inner object.

The following section of the book shows how difficult it is for Lucy as the youngest sibling to be heard, and how difficult it is for the older ones to believe she was truly in Narnia. She cannot prove it, since the portal to the other world is now closed. Instead of an entrance, there is merely the back panel of the wardrobe.

At first her siblings take her tale to be a joke, but then she is called crazy. Lucy is now doubly alone—bereft of her mother, who is far away in London, and also without the support of her siblings. She knows she has told the truth. She suffers particularly under Edmund's mocking and scorn.

The second excursion to Narnia occurs during a game of hide-and-seek between Lucy and Edmund. Edmund feels himself abandoned and becomes fearful: he is convinced that Lucy has left him alone as a kind of punishment for taunting her. In this emotionalised state, he meets the white witch. In Narnia, winter has reigned for a hundred years—caused by the tyrannical white witch Jadis, who at this time rules over Narnia. She is similar to Hans Christian Andersen's snow queen—cold and merciless, like a good mother transformed into an evil mother, with a marvellous fur coat Edmund is meant to admire: a narcissistic glorification. The white witch seduces Edmund with a magical foodstuff, Turkish delight; she recognises his greed, diverting him into absolute dependency on her. She promises to satisfy his megalomaniacal fantasies: he will become king and rule over his siblings, who will serve him. The more he eats, the less he is able to think. But after they return, Edmund leaves Lucy in the lurch, denying he has been in Narnia.

The other siblings ask the professor, who supports Lucy. Despite the prevailing doubts concerning her narrative, Lucy sticks to her inner truth. She knows she truly met the faun.

All four children take part in the third visit to Narnia. Lucy's friend, the faun, has been locked up and his house destroyed. As in many fairy tales, a bird appears who shows the children their path. The children are then cared for by a pair of beavers—mainly orally, with good food. They meet the divine lion Aslan, and fight the witch. Aslan sacrifices himself for Edmund—who becomes a traitor through Jadis—but subsequently returns from the dead. Jadis is vanquished by the children together with Aslan, whereupon the children become kings and queens of Narnia, remaining so for many years.

Aslan, the lion, embodies inner hope and goodness—internalised images of parents or good inner objects. The four siblings represent four different forms of relationship to an absent good object. Edmund feels totally abandoned, he develops paranoia, subsequently fleeing to the white witch and believing in her promises. But he is thoroughly disappointed: instead of the wonderful Turkish delight, he receives hard bread and water, and is locked away. Slowly, Edmund realises what a traitor he has been. Then, as his inner world—heretofore marked by hate and greed—begins to welcome loving thoughts, the outer reality awakens: flowers bloom, ice melts, birds start to sing.

Peter at first feels morally superior to the others. Slowly, he realises he has helped to betray Edmund, since he left Edmund alone in his own self-righteous anger. Only when he is protecting his sister Susan from a wolf does Peter come into contact with his fear and aggression. As prince, he must earn his rank. The two girls Susan and Lucy correspond to two typical female role models. When the lion withdraws, they accompany him, sharing his pain and desperation. Their empathy when they glimpse Aslan's dead body enables them to keep his greatness, his beauty, and strength alive. They have observed his demise compassionately. Owing to their perseverance, a still more powerful magic is activated, the stone table shatters, and the lion Aslan reawakens to new life. He sacrificed his life in order to save the life of traitorous Edmund. As in the story of Christ, death is also conquered. Margaret and Michael Rustin point out that "the latency child's hatred of sexuality is thus enshrined in the rules of access to Narnia" (2001, p. 53). In the later volumes, Susan, already a young woman, is not allowed to enter Narnia, since it is only open to children. Edmund is forgiven.

I will not discuss here the strongly religious themes of liberation and resurrection, since in this book we are investigating phenomena typical of latency development.

Both *Harry Potter* and the Narnia books have been filmed, and represent an important enrichment in children's literature. Children's books constitute a form of symbolic and imaginary experience, supplying a plethora of humorous, touching, and frightening scenes that the protagonists are nevertheless able to master. These books encourage readers to develop psychic space for thinking where they can recognise their feelings and become both subject and object of actions. Such books often become models for daydreams where the child herself is a protagonist in exciting dramas. These heroes and heroines who observe their own feelings and can reflect on them are valuable as examples for personal development. Symbolic representation of emotional and cognitive development goes hand in hand with a differentiated, modulated use of language.

CHAPTER FIVE

Consequences and overview

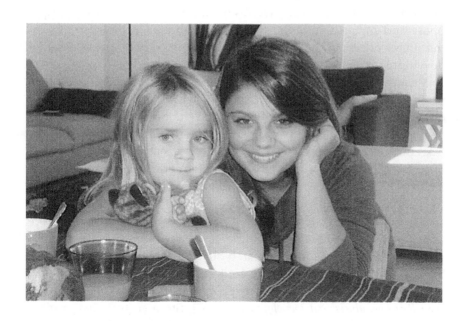

Developmental theory found its first prominent role within psychoanalytic theory. After Freud came to the revolutionary insight that real and fantasised experiences in childhood play a central role in the formation of neuroses, he attempted to reconstruct traumatising experiences through psychoanalysis. At first he thought neurotic symptoms could be traced to traumatic events in childhood, and posited a direct causal link between trauma and symptom. Accordingly, he assumed that when the patient interpreted and relived these suppressed experiences, neurosis could be altered through insight. Today, development is viewed as a non-linear process, where numerous outer and inner factors collaborate. Psychoanalysic theory still postulates that the basic pattern of the personality is structured through early experiences and that these influence our experiencing of the world, other persons, and ourselves. Freud attempted to understand psychosexual and drive developments, reconstructing through psychoanalysis the genesis of neuroses out of a patient's associations and dreams. The latency phase was long a "neglected child" (Donnellan, 1980), since Freud was more interested in the turbulent periods of psychosexual development in the Oedipal phase and puberty. Analytic work with children in their first learning phase at school, however, reveals a time of rich and variegated development.

Melanie Klein's visionary metapsychological concepts, positing a rudimentary core ego from birth on, enabled a new direction and further elaboration for Freud's developmental psychology, leading to valuable new distinctions. The quest for an object—another person—already from birth is today deemed "primary intersubjectivity" for the formation of the self, and considered a foundation for the interpretations of empirical schools. However, there are various opinions as to whether this is an inborn faculty or simply developed at a very early age. Klein speaks of an inborn rudimentary ego core and Bion of the preconception of a link between mother (nipple) and baby (mouth), whereas proponents of empirical infant research such as Daniel Stern believe the baby *acquires* the ability to make contact with the mother. In the new introduction (2010) to his *The Interpersonal World of the Infant: a View from Psychoanalysis and Development* (1985), Stern corrects his original view that intersubjectivity only originates at the age of nine months, placing it back at "practically the beginning" of life (see Bohleber, 2011, p. 772).

Klein emphasises the significance of inner reality—intrapsychic processes that result from the relationship (interpersonal dimension) between baby and mother. In her further development of psycho-analytic theory, Klein centred on the early years of life—the Oedipal phase, considered by Freud centrally important as the nucleus of neurosis. Freud considered how the Oedipal conflict is resolved to be path-setting for personality development, since the establishing of sexual orientation and the structuring of the personality is thus determined in the form of the superego. Klein concentrated attention on the baby's relationship to his mother, both in his real experience and—much more significantly—his perceptions, as altered by his fantasies, hopes, and desires, determined by the life and death drives. Theoretical and empirical (clinical) observations, developed on the mother–child matrix, supply the foundations for object relations theory, also discussed in this book.

According to object relations theory, the primary goal of the self is not drive discharge but the search for an object (the mother). Clinical work with very small children enabled Klein to support and further develop metapsychological assumptions with clinical data—for instance, her concept of the depressive and paranoid-schizoid positions, projective identification, unconscious envy, and the defence mechanism of splitting. The diversion and structuring of Oedipal triangulation in the early years of life—described by Klein as "the early stages of the Oedipus conflict"—made treatment possible for deeply disturbed psychotic patients. Her understanding of the psychotic core of early childhood and the primitive, archaic fears and defence mechanisms in children (later, in psychotic patients) was fruitfully developed both clinically and theoretically by her followers Herbert Rosenfeld, Hanna Segal, and Wilfred Bion. Clinical seminars now held for more than fifty years— led first by Betty Joseph and then Hanna Segal, Michael Feldman, John Steiner, and Ron Britton—have resulted in a close interweaving of transference interpretations, thus integrating an understanding of containment with reconstruction of the deep patterns of the personality formed in childhood (Hargreaves & Varchevker, 2004).

These concepts of early development from object relations theory constitute a shift in intellectual approach enabling recognition of deep patterns in interaction, observable in countertransference as "inner observation" and contributing to analytic interpretation. Ludwik Fleck (1935), the philosopher of science and a precursor of Thomas Kuhn

(1962), describes the necessity for special training in major scientific innovations—for instance, reading X-rays. A gradual transformation of intellectual approach is required in psychoanalytic theory, abandoning one-sided linear thought and leading to a mode of thought character-ised by interactive communication and experience within the frame-work of object relations theory. With this special training, deep layers can be revealed in clinical work, as demonstrated impressively in the London Kleinians' case studies (Britton, 1989; Feldman, 2009; Frank & Weiss, 2002; Joseph, 1989; Steiner, 1993).

Although object relations theory has always postulated a reciprocal effect between transference interpretations and the reconstruction of a life story in the here and now, it has been criticised for taking the real world into too little consideration. Thus Bohleber writes of a "declining interest on the part of psychoanalysis in questions specific to develop-ment" (2011, p. 769). The sharp criticism André Green made of empiri-cal development research has contributed to the increased distance between developmental psychology and psychoanalysis.

This book has sought particularly to show how important the con-cepts of both the early years and also of latency are, not only for child psychoanalytical practice but for anyone dealing with children and their inner worlds. The period between six and eleven years of age constitutes an important new period of life, revealing whether the par-ents' rearing of their child up to now has laid a stable foundation of self-confidence. Deeper-lying problems often become visible in latency when a child is not able to cope with the demands of school, since she is occupied with her unresolved inner fears. Case studies of children in analysis illustrate the working through and solving of these inner conflicts. With Naomi, there was a mostly loving relationship to her parents that nevertheless fell out of balance due to her parents' divorce and her father's serious illness. With Ben, the traumatic experiences he had to undergo with his drug-addicted parents had been overcome only superficially: these experiences were then manifested as learning and reading problems, requiring therapy. Only when his inner conflicts, fears, and accusations could be discussed could Ben establish an inner order enabling him to learn and acquire new knowledge. Alongside her limited intelligence, Elfi had to struggle with massive feelings of infe-riority, hidden behind the façade of a pretty, cheerful girl. The analyst's guidance and companionship enabled her to eliminate her secondary handicap (her feelings of inferiority) and give her the courage to lead a meaningful life with her limited capabilities.

Based on a thorough description of the early years of life (Diem-Wille, 2013), this book has described development in the latency period. Effects of physical growth on the body ego were described. The description of specific defence mechanisms was meant to help readers less familiar with psychoanalysis to recognise exaggerated forms of cleanliness, modesty, or precision in latency children as passing phenomena. Specific developments in feeling and thinking, as well as psychosexual development—with its influence on the child's distancing from the parents—were described in detail, in order to understand these developments as specific to latency. In children's books, forms of identification with heroes and heroines of a story were explained as experimental actions. Latency serves to stabilise identity so that the child will better handle the impending storms of adolescence. Latency thus enables a second working through and modification of early fears; the ego becomes stronger and more mature. Let me once again quote Melanie Klein as she sums up the transformations typical of latency: "The relationship to the parents is marked by great security; the introjected parents approach the image of the real parents; their standards and values, their admonishments and prohibitions are accepted and internalized, and thus Oedipal desires can be more effectively suppressed. All this represents a peak in superego development" (1952c, p. 146). Loving and restorative impulses towards parents lead to the relinquishing of incestuous desires and to progress in symbolisation. Growing ability to learn and engage in new activities (sports and hobbies) leads to an extension of interest in other persons, preparing for the choice of object in adolescence. Moral ideals are developed. When these healing tendencies are impeded by massive inner conflicts, learning problems or emotional disturbances become manifest. Through describing both normal latency children and those with emotional problems, this book has sought to aid teachers, parents, educators, and therapists in understanding the child during this phase of life.

REFERENCES

Bettelheim, B. (1976). *The Uses of Enchantment: The Meaning and Importance of Fairy Tales*. New York: Alfred A. Knopf.

Bick, E. (1968). The experience of the skin in early object-relations. *International Journal of Psychoanalysis*, *49*: 484–486. In German: Das Hauterleben in frühen Objektbeziehungen. In: G. Diem-Wille. & A. Turner (Eds.), *Ein-Blicke in die Tiefe. Die Methode der psychoanalytischen Säuglingsbeobachtung und ihre Anwendungen*. Stuttgart, Germany: Klett-Cotta, 2009. (pp. 37–40)

Bick, E. (2009). Bemerkungen zur Säuglingsbeobachtung in der psychoanalytischen Ausbildung. In: G. Diem-Wille & A. Turner (Eds.), *Ein-Blicke in die Tiefe. Die Methode der psychoanalytischen Säuglingsbeobachtung und ihre Anwendungen* (pp. 19–36). Stuttgart, Germany: Klett-Cotta.

Bion, W. R. (1957). On arrogance. *International Journal of Psychoanalysis*, *39*: 144–146. Reprinted in *Second Thoughts*. London: Karnac, 1984.

Bion, W. R. (1962). *Learning from Experience*. London: Tavistock.

Bion, W. R. (1967). A theory of thinking. In: *Second Thoughts* (pp. 93–109). London: Karnac, 1984.

Bohleber, W. (2011). Die intersubjektive Geburt des Selbst. Neue Ergebnisse der Entwicklungsforschung und ihrer Bedeutung für die Psychoanalyse, deren Behandlungstheorie und Anwendungen. Editorial in the special issue, "Wie wir wurden, was wir sind", *Subjektwerdung im Schnittpunkt von neuer Entwicklungsforschung und Psychoanalyse*, *65*: 769–777.

Bohleber, W. (2013). Editorial on: "Das Unbewusste. Metamorphosen eines Kernkonzepts". *Sonderheft Psyche, 9/10*: 807–816.

Bornstein, B. (1951). On latency. *Psychoanalytic Study of the Child, 8*: 279–285.

Brakel, L. A. W., Shevrin, H., & Villa, K. K. (2002). The priority of primary process categorizing: Experimental evidence supporting a psychoanalytic developmental hypothesis. *Journal of the American Psychoanalytic Association, 50*(2): 483–505.

Britton, R. (1989). The missing link. Parental sexuality in the Oedipus complex. In: R. Britton, M. Feldman, & E. O'Shaughnessy (Eds.), *The Oedipus Complex Today*. London: Karnac.

Brizendine, L. (2006). *The Female Brain*. New York: Morgan Road.

Brizendine, L. (2010). *The Male Brain*. New York: Three Rivers Press/Crown.

Burrison, J. A. (Ed.) (1989). *Storytellers: Folktales and Legends from the South*. Athens, GA: University of Georgia Press.

Cavell, S. (2010). *Little Did I Know. Excerpts from Memory*. Palo Alto, CA: Stanford University Press.

Churchill, W. S. (1930). *My Early Life. A Roving Commission*. London: Thornton Butterworth.

Clowes, E. (1996). Oedipal themes in latency. *Psychoanalytic Study of the Child, 51*: 436–454.

Coudenhove-Kalergi, B. (2013). *Zuhause ist überall. Erinnerungen*. Vienna: Zsolnay.

De Masi, F. (2003). Das Unbewusste und die Psychosen. *Psyche, 57*: 1–34.

Deutsch, H. (1948). *Psychology of Women, Volume I*. Boston, MA: Allyn & Bacon.

Diem-Wille, G. (2013). *The Early Years of Life*. London: Karnac.

Diem-Wille, G. (2014). Zur Bedeutung des Containments in den frühen Lebensjahren und die Bedeutung des Containments in Analysen, die Raum zum Denken eröffnen. *Kinderanalyse, 22*: 48–70.

Diem-Wille, G., & Turner, A. (2012). *Die Methode der psychoanalytischen Beobachtung. Über die Bedeutung von Containment, Identifikation, Abwehr und anderen Phänomenen in der psychoanalytischen Beobachtung*. Vienna: Facultas.

Donnellan, G. J. (1980). Conceptual models and symbol formation during the latency period. *Psychoanalytic Review, 67*: 291–312.

Erikson, E. H. (1950). *Childhood and Society*. New York: W. W. Norton.

Etchegoyen, A. (1993). Latency—a reappraisal. *International Journal of Psychoanalysis, 74*: 347–357.

Fatke, R. (2010). Introduction. In: J. Piaget: *Meine Theorie der geistigen Entwicklung*. R. Fatke (Ed.). Weinheim/Basel, Switzerland: Beltz.

Feldman, M. (1989). The Oedipus complex: manifestation in the inner world and the therapeutic situation. In: R. Britton, M. Feldman, &

E. O'Shaughnessy (Eds.), *The Oedipus Complex Today. Clinical Implications.* London: Karnac.

Feldman, M. (2009). *Doubt, Conviction and the Analytic Process. Selected Papers of Michael Feldman.* London: Routledge.

Fenichel, O. (1943). The function of children's books in latency and prepuberty periods. *Psychoanalytic Quarterly, 12*: 588–589.

Ferenczi, S. (1924). Versuch einer Genitaltheorie. In: *Schriften zur Psychoanalyse, Vol. II* (pp. 317–400). Frankfurt, Germany: S. Fischer.

Ferenczi, S. (1930). Masculine and feminine. Psychoanalytic observations on the "genital theory" and on secondary and tertiary sex characteristics. *Psychoanalytic Review, 17*(2): 105–113.

Fleck, L. (1935). *Genesis and Development of a Scientific Fact.* T. J. Trenn & R. K. Merton (Eds.). Chicago, IL: University of Chicago Press, 1979.

Franieck, L., & Günther, M. (2010). *On Latency. Individual Development, Narcissistic Impulse, Reminiscence, and Cultural Ideal.* London: Karnac.

Frank, C., & Weiss, H. (2002). *Kleinianische Theorie in klinischer Praxis. Schriften von Elizabeth Bott Spillius.* Stuttgart, Germany: Klett-Cotta.

Freud, A. (1946). *The Psychoanalytic Treatment of Children. The Writings of Anna Freud,* Vol. I. New York: International Universities Press, 1974.

Freud, S. (1900a). *The Interpretation of Dreams. S. E.,* 4–5. London: Hogarth.

Freud, S. (1901b). *The Psychopathology of Everyday Life. S. E.,* 6. London: Hogarth.

Freud, S. (1905d). *Three Essays on the Theory of Sexuality. S. E.,* 7: 125. London: Hogarth.

Freud, S. (1907c). The sexual enlightenment of children (an open letter to Dr. M. Fürst). *S. E., 9*: 129–140. London: Hogarth.

Freud, S. (1909c). Family romances. *S. E., 9*: 235. London: Hogarth.

Freud, S. (1910c). *Leonardo da Vinci and a Memory of His Childhood. S. E., 11*: 63–137. London: Hogarth.

Freud, S. (1911b). Formulations on the two principles of mental functioning. *S. E., 12*: 218–226. London: Hogarth.

Freud, S. (1914c). On narcissism: an introduction. *S. E., 14*: 69. London: Hogarth.

Freud, S. (1914g). Remembering, repeating and working-through (further recommendations on the technique of psycho-analysis, II). *S. E., 12*: 145. London: Hogarth.

Freud, S. (1919e). A child is being beaten. *S. E., 17*: 177. London: Hogarth.

Freud, S. (1920g). *Beyond the Pleasure Principle. S. E., 18*: 1–64. London: Hogarth.

Freud, S. (1923b). *The Ego and the Id. S. E., 19*: 3. London: Hogarth.

Freud, S. (1926d). *Inhibitions, Symptoms and Anxiety. S. E., 20*: 77. London: Hogarth.

Freud, S. (1933a). *New Introductory Lectures on Psycho-Analysis. S. E.*, 22: 3. London: Hogarth.

Gardner, R. W., & Moriarty, A. E. (1968). *Personality Development at Preadolescence: Explorations of Structure and Formation.* Seattle, WA: University of Washington Press.

Goldings, H. J. (1974). Jump-rope rhymes and the rhythm of latency development in girls. *Psychoanalytic Study of the Child, 29:* 431–450.

Hargreaves, E., & Varchevker, A. (2004). *In Pursuit of Psychic Change. The Betty Joseph Workshop.* Hove, UK: Brunner-Routledge.

Joseph, B. (1989). *Psychic Equilibrium and Psychic Change.* London: Routledge.

Klein, M. (1929). Infantile anxiety situations reflected in a work of art and in the creative impulse. In: *The Writings of Melanie Klein, Vol. 1* (pp. 210–218). Reprinted London: Karnac, 1975.

Klein, M. (1932). The technique of analysis in the latency period. In: *The Psychoanalysis of Children* (pp. 94–121). The International Psycho-Analytical Library. London: Hogarth.

Klein, M. (1945). The Oedipus complex in the light of early anxieties. *International Journal of Psychoanalysis, 26:* 11–33.

Klein, M. (1946). Notes on some schizoid mechanisms. In: *The Writings of Melanie Klein, Vol. 3* (pp. 1–24). Reprinted London: Karnac, 1975.

Klein, M. (1948). *Contributions to Psychoanalysis, 1921–1945.* London: Hogarth.

Klein, M. (1952c). Some theoretical conclusions regarding the emotional life of the infant. In: *The Writings of Melanie Klein, Vol. 3* (pp. 61–93). London: Hogarth and the Institute of Psychoanalysis, 1985.

Klinger, E. (1971). *Structure and Function of Fantasy.* New York: Wiley.

Kuhn, T. S. (1962). *The Structure of Scientific Revolutions.* Chicago, IL: University of Chicago Press.

Laplanche, J., & Pontalis, J. B. (1973). *The Language of Psychoanalysis.* London: Karnac, 1988.

Lewis, C. S. (1950). *The Lion, the Witch and the Wardrobe.* London: Harper Collins, 2009.

Mertens, W. (1996). *Entwicklung der Psychosexualität und der Geschlechtsidentität, Vol. II. Kindheit und Adoleszenz.* Stuttgart, Germany: Kohlhammer.

Miller, L. (1993). *Understanding Your 8 Year Old.* London: Rosendale.

Milne, A. A. (1924). *When We Were Very Young.* London: Methuen, 1992.

Milne, A. A. (1927). *Now We Are Six.* London: Methuen Children's Books, 1989.

Munro, A. (2012). Pride. In: *Dear Life.* New York: Vintage International.

Piaget, J. (1926). *La representation du monde chez l 'enfant.* Paris: Presses Universitaires de France.

Piaget, J. (1964). *Theorien und Methoden der modernen Erziehung*. Vienna: Molden, 1972. (Originally published as: *Psychologie et Pédagogie. Six Etudes de Psychologie*. Paris: Société Nouvelle des Éditions Gouthier.)

Piaget, J. (1983). *Meine Theorie der geistigen Entwicklung*. R. Fatke (Ed.). Weinheim/Basel, Switzerland: Beltz, 2010.

Pikler, F. (2001). *Lasst mir Zeit. Die selbständige Bewegungsentwicklung des Kindes bis zum freien Gehen*. Munich, Germany: Pflaum.

Renton, A. (2014). The abusers could still be teaching. In: *The Guardian Weekly*, May 23: 26–29.

Riesenberg-Malcolm, R. (2001). Bion's theory of containment. In: C. Bronstein (Ed.), *Kleinian Theory. A Contemporary Perspective* (pp. 165–180). London: Whurr.

Rosenfeld, H. (1987). *Impasse and Interpretation*. London: Tavistock.

Rowling, J. K. (1997). *Harry Potter and the Philosopher's Stone*. London: Bloomsbury.

Rustin, M. (2008). Some historical and theoretical observations. In: M. Rustin & J. Bradley (Eds.), *Work Discussion. Learning from Reflective Practice in Work with Children and Families* (pp. 3–21). London: Karnac.

Rustin, M., & Rustin, M. (2001). The inner world of Harry Potter. In: *Narratives of Love and Loss. Studies in Modern Children's Fiction*. London: Karnac.

Salzberger-Wittenberg, I., Henry-Williams, G., & Osborne, E. (1997). *Die Pädagogik der Gefühle. Emotionale Aspekte beim Lernen und Lehren*. Vienna: Wiener Universitätsverlag.

Sarnoff, C. A. (1976). *Latency*. New York: Jason Aronson.

Spillius, E. B. (1988). Introduction to "A Theory of Thinking." In: *Melanie Klein Today: Developments in Theory and Practice*. London: Tavistock/ Routledge.

Spillius, E. B. (2011). *The New Dictionary of Kleinian Thought*. London: Routledge.

Steiner, J. (1993). *Psychic Retreats. Pathological Organizations in Psychotic, Neurotic and Borderline Patients*. London: Routledge.

Stern, D. N. (1985). *The Interpersonal World of the Infant: a View from Psychoanalysis and Development*. New York: Basic Books, 2010.

Strouhal, M. (2014). *Konflikterleben in Bildungseinrichtungen aus psychoanalytischer Sicht*. Master's dissertation in psychoanalytic observational studies, University of Klagenfurt, Austria.

Wagner-Schick, U. (2000). *Die Förderklasse—eine "pädagogische Intensivstation" für verhaltensauffällige Kinder?* Diploma thesis, University of Vienna.

Weiss, H. (2013). Unbewusste Phantasien als strukturierende Prinzipien und Organisatoren des psychischen Lebens. In: "Psyche, Das

Unbewusste. Metamorphosen eines Kernkonzepts". *Sonderheft Psyche*, *9/10*: 903–930.

Winnicott, D. W. (1956). Primary maternal preoccupation. In: *Through Paediatrics to Psycho-Analysis* (pp. 300–305). London: Hogarth, 1975.

Winnicott, D. W. (1958). Child analysis in latency years. In: *The Maturational Processes and the Facilitating Environment: Studies in the Theory of Emotional Development* (pp. 115–123). The International Psycho-Analytical Library. London: Hogarth and the Institute of Psychoanalysis, 1965.

Winnicott, D. W. (1963). The development of the capacity for concern In: *The Maturational Processes and the Facilitating Environment: Studies in the Theory of Emotional Development* (pp. 64–73). The International Psycho-Analytical Library. London: Hogarth and the Institute of Psychoanalysis, 1965.

Winnicott, D. W. (1965). *The Maturational Processes and the Facilitating Environment: Studies in the Theory of Emotional Development*. London: Hogarth.

Zulliger, H. (1970). *Heilende Kräfte im kindlichen Spiel*. Stuttgart, Germany: Fischer.

Zwettler-Otte, S. (2002). Harry Potter und die Bausteine eines Welterfolgs. In: *Von Robinson bis Harry Potter. Kinderbuch-Klassiker psychoanalytisch*. Munich, Germany: dtv.

INDEX

Names